THE MENTAL STATUS
EXAMINATION IN
NEUROLOGY

THE MENTAL STATUS EXAMINATION IN NEUROLOGY

FOURTH EDITION

Richard L. Strub, MD
Chairman, Department of Neurology
Ochsner Clinic
Clinical Professor of Neurology
Tulane University
New Orleans, Louisiana

F. William Black, PhD
Professor of Psychiatry and Neurology
Director, Neuropsychology Laboratory
Tulane University Medical Center
New Orleans, Louisiana

Foreword by Norman Geschwind

Illustrations by Ann Strub

F. A. DAVIS COMPANY • Philadelphia

F. A. Davis Company
1915 Arch Street
Philadelphia, PA 19103

Printed in the United States of America

Last digit indicates print number: 10 9 8 7 6 5 4 3

Senior Medical Editor: Robert W. Reinhardt
Senior Developmental Editor: Bernice M. Wissler
Production Editor: Michael Schnee
Cover Designer: Louis J. Forgione

As new scientific information becomes available through basic and clinical research, recommended treatments and drug therapies undergo changes. The authors and publisher have done everything possible to make this book accurate, up to date, and in accord with accepted standards at the time of publication. The authors, editors, and publisher are not responsible for errors or omissions or for consequences from application of the book, and make no warranty, expressed or implied, with regard to the contents of the book. Any practice described in this book should be applied by the reader in accordance with professional standards of care used with regard to the unique circumstances that may apply in each situation. The reader is advised always to check product information (package inserts) for changes and new information regarding dose and contraindications before administering any drug. Caution is especially urged when using new or infrequently ordered drugs.

Library of Congress Cataloging-in-Publication Data

Strub, Richard L., 1939–
    The mental status examination in neurology / Richard L. Strub, F.
  William Black : foreword by Norman Geschwind : illustrations by Ann
  Strub. — 4th ed.
      p.   cm.
  Includes bibliographical references and index.
  ISBN 0-8036-0427-0 (alk. paper)
    1. Mental status examination.   2. Neurobehavioral disorders—
  Diagnosis. I. Black, F. William. II. Title.
    [DNLM: 1. Neurologic Examination.   2. Delirium, Dementia,
  Amnestic, Cognitive Disorders—diagnosis.   3. Nervous System
  Diseases—diagnosis.   4. Neuropsychological Tests.   WL 141 S925m
  1999]
  RC386.6.M44S87   2000
  616.8'0475—dc21
  DNLM/DLC
  for Library of Congress   99-24985
                                                CIP

FOREWORD

The testing of mental status has a curious, not to say anomalous, position in the examination of patients. Every medical student has had the experience of being given a long and detailed outline, or an even longer booklet, containing a seemingly endless list of items. Even if he should go to the trouble of memorizing these miniature compendia, he is likely to discover that his teachers, both neurologic and psychiatric, are disinclined to be concerned with the detailed examination, and often rely, at best, on fragments. The examinations themselves seem to differ from those in other fields of medicine. The student rapidly comes to appreciate the direct relevance of rectal tenderness to the diagnosis of appendicitis or of pulsus paradoxus to pericardial effusion. The mental examination seems to him to be much more indirectly and diffusely related to diagnostic categories.

Equally striking, or even more so, is the usual lack of direct correlation between the test items and disorders of structure or physiology. Orthopnea, swollen neck veins, rales at the lung bases, cardiac enlargement, characteristic murmurs, and auricular fibrillation not only mean congestive failure, but all the findings on examination come to blend almost imperceptibly and effortlessly with knowledge of normal cardiac structures and physiology and awareness of lawful derangements in disease. This easy understanding of the relationship of abnormal findings on examination to anatomy and physiology seems to be lacking in the mental examination.

There is, however, no reason that this situation should persist. The growth of knowledge concerning disorders of the higher functions has been rapid over the past quarter century. Not only has our ability to specify anatomic systems involved in different behaviors increased, but even more important, we have come to a deeper understanding of the mechanisms underlying disordered function.

This book, therefore, represents a valuable synthesis. For the attentive reader, it will yield important advantages. Not only does it shift the emphasis to those methods of examination that have proven their worth in the clinic but it provides wherever possible a link to known anatomic and physiologic mechanisms.

Several final comments are appropriate. There is a widespread, usually tacit but often openly expressed, view that mental examination is a long and arduous task. Most physicians have learned that although a "complete" survey of the heart, lungs, abdomen, and other structures can take hours, intimate knowledge of the examination and repeated practice enable them to obtain essential information in a very brief time. Those who have learned the mental examination and have practiced it often can equally well obtain vital information rapidly and efficiently when necessary. There is another common view that mental examination can be handed over to others. We should remember, however, that the real measure of a physician's usefulness lies in his capacity to make critical decisions when he is alone with the patient in the small hours of the night. Furthermore, unless he can screen patients effectively, he will fail to refer intelligently to others. Finally, if the ultimate decisions lie in his hands, he will fail to use adequately the opinions of his consultants unless he has a basic understanding of all aspects of his patient's problems. The newer knowledge of mental examination set forth within this book is essential not merely to the neurologist or psychiatrist, but to all physicians.

Norman Geschwind, MD
James Jackson Putnam Professor of Neurology
Harvard Medical School
1977

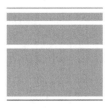

PREFACE

The basic purpose and scope of this book have not changed since the first edition was published in 1977. In the intervening years, we have gained considerable additional clinical experience with the mental status examination and have standardized most of its sections. Some of the standardized items have been compared with the objective data generated from formal neuropsychological tests. These comparisons have been very rewarding because the mental status examination has been proved an accurate and valid method for identifying and diagnosing organic brain disease as well as for describing relative levels of functioning. Age-related norms are presented for most aspects of the examination. These data are important because we have found that our patients aged 70 and older do perform less adequately on some of the critical items, especially new learning, than do the younger patients. This difference is important to take into account when assessing the elderly for early dementia. False positive results can occur and must be minimized.

In the first edition, we assured the reader that after reading and using the book he or she would be able to perform a brief screening examination. It has been suggested that we provide more concrete guidelines for tailoring the examination for brief administration. Therefore, in the summary section of this edition, we have included some ways to use the examination as a screening procedure, particularly in the extremely important areas of diagnosing dementia and differentiating between organic and functional disorders. A shortened form of the examination is presented, with standardization for normals of various ages and for patients with Alzheimer's disease.

We have updated the references in all chapters; this is particularly the case in those sections in which new studies have refined the neuroanatomic and neuropsychological aspects of cognitive functions. The section on neuropsychological testing has been fully revised to include a survey of the most commonly used tests, to drop some tests that have fallen from general use, and to make this section more clinically relevant to both physicians and other health-care providers and to psychologists.

In general, we feel that the earlier editions were good and have demonstrated their value in widespread clinical use. With each edition we have tried to refine both the process of the examination and its clinical usefulness. We hope this text will prove as useful to others who are interested in neurobehavior as it has been to our students, residents, and professional colleagues.

RL Strub, MD
FW Black, PhD
New Orleans, LA

CONTENTS

THE MENTAL STATUS EXAMINATION: A RATIONALE AND OVERVIEW

Human behavior is extremely complex and multifaceted. Because of its complexity, it is not surprising that brain disease or dysfunction can significantly affect a patient's behavior in a variety of ways. Understanding this behavioral disruption caused by brain disease is a substantial and often frustrating problem for the clinician faced with the tasks of diagnosis and management. Patients with organically related changes in cognitive or emotional behavior have often fallen just outside the limits of traditional psychiatry and neurology. These borderline cognitive behavior changes have long been called **organic brain syndromes**, a general term that covers any possible behavior change resulting from brain damage or dysfunction. In the American Psychiatric Association's *Diagnostic and Statistical Manual of Mental Disorders, Fourth Edition (DSM-IV),*[1] such conditions are categorized as delirium, dementia, and amnestic and other cognitive disorders. The *DSM-IV* classifies noncognitive behavior changes, such as the personality disorder seen in patients with frontal lobe disease, as mental disorders due to a general medical condition. Neurologists now use the term **neurobehavioral disorders** to include both cognitive and noncognitive organically based behavior changes.

In the past several decades, particularly because of the focus on Alzheimer's disease, there has been a renewed interest in these organic syndromes. It is now possible, owing to a greater understanding of these conditions, to relate particular behavioral deficit patterns to specific diseases and to damage in particular regions of the brain.

The magnitude and social impact of these neurobehavioral disorders are enormous. These disorders are very common in the hospital and office practices of primary care physicians, neurologists, and psychiatrists. In clinical

1

practice, dementia, aphasia, and confusional states (delirium) are very commonly encountered. Primary organic brain disease accounted for at least 30% of all first admissions to psychiatric hospitals in the 1950s,[2] and this incidence is increasing.[3] Dementia is now the fourth leading cause of death in the adult population in the United States, a trend that can only worsen as the lifespan increases. Students should now be able to recognize the signs of early dementia as readily as they do those of acquired immune deficiency syndrome (AIDS) or congestive heart failure.

For examiners to understand organically based behavior changes adequately and to apply this understanding to individual clinical cases, they must use a systematic behavioral examination called the **mental status examination**, *an orderly assessment of the important cognitive and emotional functions that are commonly and characteristically disturbed in patients with organic brain disease.*

WHEN SHOULD A MENTAL STATUS EXAMINATION BE PERFORMED?

Because the mental status examination is not always included in a routine neurologic evaluation, it is important that the clinician be able to determine when inclusion of the mental status examination is appropriate. Just as the patient with otitis externa does not routinely require an electrocardiogram, the patient with a peripheral neuropathy does not usually need a full mental status examination. Conversely, any patient who complains of memory or other cognitive difficulties should receive a comprehensive mental status examination, just as the patient with a fever, headache, and stiff neck requires an immediate computed tomography (CT) scan and lumbar puncture.

Known Brain Lesions

Full mental status testing is definitely indicated for many patients. Patients with *known brain lesions* such as tumors, trauma, or vascular accident should have an initial screening mental status evaluation to document any cognitive or emotional changes. Even with the current state of neurobehavioral knowledge, subtle behavioral deficits secondary to brain lesions are sometimes overlooked by the treating physician. Many patients with mild aphasias or memory deficits after craniotomy, increased irritability and decreased ability to concentrate after head trauma, or marked emotional lability after infectious neurologic disease are released from the hospital without adequate recognition of these cognitive and emotional deficits. Such patients frequently become emotionally frustrated, have difficulty with social readjustment, and are unable to carry out the routine demands of home and vocation. Early recognition of the neurobehavioral sequelae of known brain lesions helps the physician explain the totality of the patient's disability to the family and employers. This prevents needless frustration on the patient's part, as well as misunderstanding of the patient's behavior by family members. Such documentation helps immeasurably in planning social and vocational rehabilitation when indicated.

Suspected Brain Lesions

Another large group of patients requiring mental status testing consists of *those in whom a brain lesion is suspected* because of recent onset of seizures, headaches, behavior change, or head trauma. Brain tumors, subdural hematomas, small infarcts, or cerebral atrophy may go undetected on the routine neurologic examination, whereas the cognitive effects of these lesions are often readily apparent on a complete mental status examination. We have seen a 46-year-old man who was admitted to the infectious disease isolation unit because of fever, jumbled speech, and confusion. His admitting diagnosis was "probable encephalitis." Mental status testing the morning after admission revealed an aphasia rather than a confusional state. Because the finding of aphasia is almost pathognomonic of significant left hemisphere disease, a left carotid arteriogram was performed and a large subdural hematoma found. With appropriate treatment (surgery), the patient had an uneventful and complete recovery. Because of the widespread use of noninvasive neuroimaging techniques, particularly CT and magnetic resonance imaging (MRI), it is now much less likely that a mass lesion would remain undetected in such a setting; in patients in whom the diagnosis of neurologic disease is equivocal, however, the mental status examination can be as specific in documenting a brain lesion and indicating its location as the elicitation of Babinski's sign.

Psychiatric Patients

A full mental status examination should be performed on *all psychiatric patients*, particularly those whose psychiatric symptoms have appeared rather acutely and are superimposed on a life history of normal emotional functioning. Patients with organic brain disease frequently initially present with emotional and behavioral changes and come first to the attention of the family physician or consulting psychiatrist.[3] This presentation is especially characteristic of frontal and temporal tumors, hydrocephalus, or cortical atrophy.

The most common emotional change seen in such patients is depression; therefore, *brain disease should be strongly suspected in any patient with a middle- or late-life depression that is not clearly related to a recent emotional or social crisis* (i.e., adjustment disorder with depressed mood). In our clinical practice, we have seen a number of patients being treated for an apparent depressive illness who have, in fact, demonstrated signs of primary organic disease on mental status testing and subsequent neurodiagnostic procedures (e.g., CT, MRI, and neuropsychologic evaluation).

Although the differentiation between psychiatric and organic disease is critically important, unfortunately it is sometimes difficult and not always possible. The functionally depressed patient with psychomotor retardation may perform poorly on some aspects of the mental status examination and in this way superficially present the picture of a true dementia rather than a pseudodementia. Other patients have elements of both organic and functional disease; for example, patients with early Alzheimer's dementia often present with significant associated depression or anxiety. At times, considerable effort is required to separate the respective components, even on careful clinical examination. The mental status examination is not infallible, even in the hands of an experienced examiner. The fact remains, however, that most of these patients with combined problems can be correctly classified if appropriate mental testing is done.

Vague Behavioral Complaints

A final group of patients in whom mental status screening is extremely important is *those who initially present, or are brought in by their families, with vague behavioral complaints* that are difficult clinically to substantiate and quantify on standard neurologic examination.

Complaints such as memory problems, difficulty in concentration, declining interest in family or work, and various physical complaints having no obvious organic etiology should alert the clinician to the possibility of organic brain disease. The determination of the etiology of such problems involves a difficult but important differentiation among functional, neurologic, and other medical causes. Again, this can often be best accomplished with the aid of data provided by the mental status examination.

HOW SHOULD A MENTAL STATUS EXAMINATION BE PERFORMED?

Just as with any comprehensive medical examination, mental status testing must be arranged systematically. The mental status examination differs somewhat in that *it must be performed in a hierarchic manner*, beginning with the most basic function—level of consciousness—and proceeding through the basic cognitive functions (e.g., language, constructions) to the more complex areas of verbal reasoning and calculating ability.

When the patient shows impaired performance on early sections of the examination (e.g., in language), it is difficult, if not impossible, for the examiner to assess accurately verbal memory (an extremely important function) or any other function that requires language. Similarly, the inattentive patient will miss important details during much of the higher-level testing, especially on memory and calculation items. If the mental status examination is performed in a haphazard manner, without regard for the hierarchic nature of cognitive performance, erroneous conclusions can be drawn.

The mental status examination as presented in this book may seem exceptionally detailed, and it may appear that the examination would take hours to complete in its entirety. This conception is similar to the beginning clinician's first attempts to understand the evaluation of the cranial nerves or the brachial plexus. When first learning to administer the examination, it is wise to evaluate several patients fully, to gain experience in performing and interpreting all test items. With time, the examination can be completed relatively rapidly (within 15 to 30 minutes) and will yield considerable valuable data. In Chapter 10, we have summarized the examination and indicated ways to tailor it to meet the demands of time and of specific patients.

In many cases, a brief examination will provide sufficient definitive data to allow the correct diagnosis and appropriate medical treatment. As an example of the ease of administering a meaningful examination in a brief period of time, a psychiatrist, called in the middle of the night to see a patient who was "talking out of his head," started to examine the patient's language and found that the patient was actually aphasic and not psychotic. At this point, the psychiatrist consulted with a neurologist, who admitted the patient to the neurology service rather than to the psychiatric unit. In this case, the psychiatrist had properly evaluated the patient and averted an inappropriate type of hospitalization and treatment. We were called to see a similar case, in which a young man had been admitted to the psychiatric service because he was answering all questions inappropriately and did not make sense in conversation. This behavior had initially disturbed his parents, who had brought him to the emergency room. On evaluation, the patient had little, if any, comprehension of language and was producing fluent paraphasic speech (aphasia). An MRI scan revealed a large hematoma in the dominant temporal lobe. His apparent "craziness" was due to a readily diagnosed organic disorder, and his psychiatric hospitalization had resulted from the admitting physician's lack of recognition of the patient's actual condition. In this case, demonstration of a typical pattern of aphasia not only indicated the presence of organic disease, but also strongly suggested the location of the lesion.

These examples illustrate that even a brief examination by a skilled examiner can be of critical clinical importance for some patients. Other patients, however, may require a more comprehensive assessment. The patient who is referred after a head injury requires a detailed elucidation of cognitive strengths and deficits to allow for appropriate social and vocational rehabilitation. This need for a comprehensive mental status examination is amply demonstrated in the following case. The physical medicine service requested a consultation on a 32-year-old woman who had suffered a severe basilar skull fracture several months previously and was not progressing satisfactorily in the inpatient rehabilitation program. The staff also noted her "difficult" and "uncooperative" behavior. Mental status testing revealed an apathetic patient without insight or concern, who had moderately impaired attention. Multiple significant cognitive deficits were demonstrated, including a mild generalized dementia, moderately impaired recent and remote memory, severely impaired new-learning ability, and a moderate to severe impairment of all higher-level cognitive functions (abstraction, calculations, and so forth). The documentation of an organic behavior change and significant cognitive deficits explained both the patient's difficult ward behavior and her inability to participate fully in a demanding rehabilitation program. Her program was restructured and her treatment goals were altered relative to the limitations caused by her cognitive and behavioral deficits.

In complicated situations, when extensive and quantitative data regarding cognitive and emotional functioning are required for proper patient management, consultation should be obtained from relevant ancillary professionals. These frequently include neuropsychologists and speech pathologists. *The bedside or office mental status examination as outlined in this book is very effective for diagnosing organic disease and for evaluating major areas of deficit.* By its nature, the examination is *qualitative* and does not offer the advantages of standardized quantitative data, which are necessary in evaluating subtle deficits, planning for comprehensive rehabilitation efforts, and assessing improvements in levels of functioning. The neuropsychologist can provide these data and additional valuable consultation whenever a definitive evaluation is required. Discharge planning and vocational or educational re-entry are also greatly aided by the findings of a comprehensive neuropsychologic assessment.

For patients with significant communication problems, referral to a speech pathologist is important for comprehensive evaluation of language, possible treatment, and counseling to facilitate communication between the patient and other family members. Chapter 11 deals in detail with the specifics of the consultation process.

REFERENCES

1. American Psychiatric Association: Diagnostic and Statistical Manual of Mental Disorders, ed 4 (DSM-IV). American Psychiatric Association, Washington, DC, 1994.
2. Malzberg, B: Important statistical data about mental illness. In Arieti, S (ed): American Handbook of Psychiatry, Vol 1. Basic Books, New York, 1959, pp 161–174.
3. Strub, RL: Mental disorders in brain disease. In Vinken PJ, Bruyn, GW, and Klawans, HL (eds): Handbook of Clinical Neurology, Vol 2, Neurobehavioral Disorders. Elsevier, New York, 1985, pp 413–441.

HISTORY AND BEHAVIORAL OBSERVATIONS

Most sections of the mental status examination involve the evaluation of specific cognitive functions such as memory and language. Before beginning formal testing, however, the examiner must obtain a clinical history and make specific observations regarding the patient's physical appearance, mood, and behavior. These observations provide important information for the interpretation of data from subsequent parts of the examination.

HISTORY

The history should be directed toward four primary areas of clinical concern. First, *the presence or absence of the classic behavioral changes indicative of organic dysfunction* (e.g., memory impairment or language disorder) must be established. Second, *the possibility of both adjustment and functional psychiatric disorders* must be considered. Although this book is primarily concerned with the changes in emotions and behavior that are seen as a result of organic brain disease, the consideration of classic psychiatric syndromes is important for several specific reasons:

1. At times, a specific lesion of the brain (e.g., a tumor of the left frontal lobe) may produce a clinical picture that is superficially indistinguishable from that of a major functional illness.[26,27] Diagnoses of depression or mania, schizophrenia, and personality disorders have all been described in patients with brain disease. These diagnoses are classified in the *DSM-IV*[1] respectively as mood disorder, psychotic disorder, and personality change due to a general medical condition (not substance-induced).

2. Patients with primary organic disease also commonly develop associated or secondary emotional symptoms such as depression, anxiety, or paranoia.

3. Another important area in which the symptomatology of organic disease and that of emotional disorders overlaps is pseudodementia, a condition in which the patient has symptoms and mental status findings that initially suggest a diagnosis of dementia but eventually prove to be secondary to depression, anxiety, or other psychiatric disorders.

4. Some patients with a major psychiatric disease (e.g., schizophrenia) will demonstrate cognitive deficits on the mental status examination. This may be due to a concomitant acquired brain lesion or may, in fact, be a part of the total clinical picture of these diseases. The incidence of cognitive dysfunction in nonfamilial schizophrenic patients is substantially higher than expected. When significant cognitive deficits are found in psychiatric patients, a neurodiagnostic evaluation including a mental status examination should be conducted.

The third focus of the history is to establish *the patient's premorbid behavior and level of functioning.* Information such as education and vocational history are important for establishing expected levels of functioning on the mental status examination. For example, the patient with a third-grade education and an inconsistent low-level work history would not be expected to perform at a high level on arithmetic or abstract reasoning tests.

The fourth area of importance is *the patient's general medical status.* Many medical conditions such as endocrine diseases, chronic renal or hepatic disorders, acquired immune deficiency syndrome (AIDS), and chronic alcohol or drug abuse adversely affect mental functioning. In some instances, particularly in elderly individuals, the use of multiple prescription and nonprescription medications can also deleteriously affect mental status.[16] When such conditions do affect mental functioning, they usually produce a confusional state, but they may mimic a dementia, depression, or other mental disorder. It is very important to diagnose these conditions early, when they are often completely reversible.

History Outline

The following elements in the history are particularly important in evaluating a patient with behavior change. Because such patients may not be able to provide a complete and accurate history, it is prudent to obtain the initial information from a family member or other individual who is very familiar with the patient. Even if the patient is able to give a history, corroborative information from a second source is advisable to ensure accuracy.

1. Description of present illness
   A. Nature and date of onset
   B. Duration of illness
   C. Description of behavioral change associated with illness
2. Other relevant organic behavioral symptoms
   A. Unusual or bizarre behavior (e.g., nocturnal wandering)
   B. Evidence of poor social judgment (e.g., discarding new clothes in the trash or being verbally abusive at social gatherings without provocation); this information should be obtained from someone other than the patient
   C. Attention and concentration problems
   D. Language problems (e.g., word-finding difficulty, comprehension deficits, or tangential verbal responses)
   E. Reading, writing, or calculation difficulty (e.g., inability to balance checkbook)
   F. Memory difficulty (recent and remote)
   G. Difficulty with geographic orientation (i.e., getting lost)
   H. Trouble driving or carrying out simple activities such as using the microwave or TV remote control.
3. Psychiatric symptoms
   A. Paranoia
   B. Hallucinations
   C. Delusions
   D. Depression
   E. Anxiety, agitation, or violence
   F. Other
4. Past history
   A. Previous neurologic disease or psychiatric problems
   B. Other medical disease
   C. Drug and alcohol use and abuse
   D. Use of prescription medications and over-the-counter medications
   E. Head trauma (comment on severity)
   F. Seizures
   G. Central nervous system infections
   H. Toxic exposure
5. Birth and developmental history
   A. Brain damage from birth
   B. Developmental delays
      (1) Motor
      (2) Language
      (3) Intellectual
      (4) Academic
      (5) Emotional or social

6. Educational and vocational history
   A. Highest school grade attained
   B. Adequacy as a student
   C. Vocation
      (1) Types of jobs
      (2) Frequency of job changes
      (3) Recent problems with job
7. Family history
   A. Neurologic or psychiatric disease in other family members
   B. Familial neurologic disease (e.g., Huntington's disease, Alzheimer's disease)
   C. Familial predilection for a particular disease process that may involve the central nervous system (e.g., hypertension and stroke)

BEHAVIORAL OBSERVATION

The primary purpose of this section is to provide a formal framework to assist the examiner both in systematically observing behavior and obtaining reliable and valid reports on the patient's behavior from other observers, such as the spouse, children, and so on. A careful observation and report of behavior is important because:

1. Several specific neurobehavioral syndromes (e.g., acute confusional state [delirium], frontal lobe syndrome, and the denial-neglect syndromes) are diagnosed primarily on the basis of their behavioral manifestations.

2. Such observations provide crucial data to aid in the differential diagnosis between organic and functional disorders.

3. A significant behavioral disturbance may dramatically interfere with subsequent formal testing (e.g., a patient in an organic confusional state will perform poorly on memory testing because of inattention).

The discussions of behavior in this chapter are primarily concerned with the identification and description of organic disease (physical brain disease) and its effects. Extensive discussions of behavior from a psychiatric viewpoint are included in all major psychiatric texts (e.g., references 2, 13, 18, and 24). See also Trzepacz and Baker[31] for a thorough presentation of a comprehensive psychiatrically oriented mental status examination.

Physical Appearance

Many patients with either brain disease or functional disorders show *characteristic patterns of physical appearance*. Classic examples range from that of the patient with unilateral neglect who exhibits a total lack of attention to dress and care (e.g., shaving and washing) one side of the body, to that of the obsessive-compulsive patient who may be scrupulously groomed and unnecessarily fastidious in matters relating to cleanliness and manner. Obvious neurologic signs such as hemiplegia or chorea are not specifically mentioned in this text. The following aspects of appearance should be noted:

1. General appearance
   A. Descriptive data
      (1) Age
      (2) Height and weight
   B. General impression of appearance
      (1) Appearance for chronologic age
      (2) Posture
      (3) Facial expression
      (4) Eye contact
2. Personal cleanliness
   A. Skin
   B. Hair
   C. Nails
   D. Teeth
   E. Beard
   F. Indications of unilateral neglect
3. Habits of dress
   A. Type of clothing
   B. Cleanliness of clothing
   C. Sloppiness in dressing
   D. Excessive fastidiousness in dressing and grooming
   E. Indications of unilateral neglect
4. Motor activity
   A. Level of general activity
      (1) Placid versus tense
      (2) Hyperkinetic versus hypokinetic
      (3) Evidence of psychomotor retardation (seen in the subcortical dementias of AIDS, progressive supranuclear palsy, and so on)
   B. Abnormal posturing
      (1) Tics
      (2) Facial grimaces
      (3) Bizarre gestures
      (4) Other involuntary movements

Mood and General Emotional Status

Mood is the prevailing and conscious emotional feeling expressed by the patient. **Emotional status** is a general term to indicate the patient's behavior; it may be evaluated through direct observation of the patient during the examination. Certain brain diseases (e.g., frontal lobe disease), as well as some psychiatric conditions, may be distinguished by rather characteristic distur-bances of mood and emotional status. Such disturbances may adversely affect performance on subsequent portions of the mental status examination. The following outline is intended not to be a complete and definitive psychiatric examination but rather to provide a framework for the brief assessment of emotional status.

1. Mood
    A. Normal for the situation
    B. Sadness (hopelessness, grief, or loss)
    C. Elation (inappropriate optimism or boastfulness)
    D. Apathy and lack of concern
    E. Constancy or fluctuations in mood
    F. Inappropriate mood: expressed affect inconsistent with the content of thought
2. Emotional status
    A. Degree of cooperation with examiner
    B. Anxiety
    C. Depression
    D. Suspiciousness
    E. Anger and/or hostility
    F. Specific inappropriate emotional responses to particular situations
    G. Reality testing
        (1) Delusions (false beliefs)
        (2) Illusions (misperceptions of real stimuli)
        (3) Hallucinations
        (4) Paranoid thinking
    H. Indications of specific nonpsychotic emotional symptoms
        (1) Phobias
        (2) Chronic anxiety (generalized or specific)
        (3) Obsessive-compulsive thinking, behavior, or both
        (4) Depression
        (5) Mania
        (6) Somatic preoccupation
        (7) Dissociative symptoms
    I. Abnormalities in language or speech
        (1) Neologisms (personal formation of a new word without real meaning except to the patient)
        (2) Flight of ideas in thinking and speaking
        (3) Loose associations in thinking and speaking

Clinical Syndromes

Several distinct clinical entities are recognized primarily through behavioral observation rather than by specific cognitive testing. These syndromes primarily involve disturbances in mood, personality, and emotional reaction more than alterations in cognition. The diagnosis, therefore, is made by systematic behavioral observation.

Acute Confusional State (Delirium)

The most common of the neurologically based behavioral syndromes seen in a general hospital population is the **acute confusional state** (also known as delirium or toxic-metabolic encephalopathy). The acute confusional state has a characteristic constellation of behavioral and historical findings. The onset of symptoms is usually fairly acute, appearing over hours or days.

Generally, *the most reliable clinical feature distinguishing the acute confusional state from other organic or functional disorders is a clouding of consciousness.* Although this term may seem somewhat vague, it does accurately describe the mental state of the confused patient. Specifically, **clouding of consciousness** refers to both a dulling of cognitive processes and a general impairment of alertness.[25] These patients are inattentive and produce incoherent conversations that drift from the central point; they are inconsistent and confabulatory in reporting recent events (e.g., patients may tell the examiner that they have just come back from a walk with a friend when, in fact, they have been in their hospital bed for the entire day); and they often demonstrate fluctuations in their level of consciousness. Hallucinations (often visual) and agitation are often present. Patients who are grossly confusional may be severely agitated and shout incoherently; these patients usually require restraints to prevent them from disrupting intravenous lines, urinary catheters, and other apparatus. Patients with mild confusion may appear normal superficially, but on systematic examination may demonstrate mild degrees of inattention and disorientation and may have difficulty holding a coherent conversation. On specific questioning, they may admit to nocturnal hallucinations and delusions. Confusional behavior is rarely stable, characteristically waxing and waning throughout the day and night. At night, when environmental stimuli are reduced, the confusion and agitation often become accentuated.

The confusional state is a very important abnormal behavioral pattern to recognize because it is usually the behavioral manifestation of an acute medical problem rather than of a neurologic or psychiatric condition. Toxic reactions to drugs or drug withdrawal, sepsis, metabolic imbalance, or early heart, pulmonary, or hepatic failure are common causes. Postoperative confusional behavior is also extremely common. In general, elderly patients, especially those with signs of early dementia, are the most likely to develop confusional states in the aforementioned medical situations.[11,15,22]

We have developed a delirium scale (Table 2–1) that can be particularly useful to house officers when they are first exposed to confusional patients. This scale consists of the most common clinical features of the confusional state. The examiner must determine the presence or absence of each feature

TABLE 2-1. **Delirium Scale Scoresheet***				
History				
1. Speed of onset of behavior change	3	2		0
2. Fluctuation over 24 hours	3		1	0
3. Sleep-wake disturbances	3		1	0
4. Hallucinations (visual or tactile)	3			0
5. Inappropriate behavior	3	2	1	0
Clinical Features				
6. Level of consciousness	3	2	1	0
7. Psychomotor activity level	3	2	1	0
8. Incoherence and disorganization	3	2	1	0
9. Attention	3	2	1	0
10. Intelligibility of speech	3	2	1	0
11. Misinterpretation of surroundings	3	2	1	0
12. Orientation	3	2	1	0
a. Time: Year Month Date Day Season				
b. Place: State Town County Hospital Floor				
Scale: (3) 9–10, (2) 6–8, (1) 3–5, (0) 0–2				
13. Construction ability—clock drawing	3	2	1	0
Total (39 maximum)				

*3 is normal; 0 is grossly abnormal.

and judge its severity based on several variables. This scale has proved clinically reliable and valid and is useful in differentiating delirium from dementia (Fig. 2–1).

Although psychiatrists or neurologists are often asked to see these patients because of their abnormal behavior or change in mental status, most patients require primary medical treatment in addition to medication for behavioral control. The confusional state may linger for many days, even after initiating appropriate medical treatment; during this period tranquilizers may be used to calm the patient's agitation.

The confusional state usually results from widespread cortical and subcortical neuronal dysfunction. Cortical dysfunction causes an alteration in the content of consciousness, whereas involvement of the ascending activating system leads to the disturbances of basic arousal. With focal brain disease, confusional behavior may also be seen. This is particularly true in the first few days after an acute cerebrovascular accident (especially where medial temporal lobe or inferior parietal or prefrontal cortex is involved) or in patients who have brain tumors with associated increased intracranial pressure.

Further mental status testing results are adversely affected in patients in a confusional state. Owing to inattention and general cortical dysfunction, patients cannot perform adequately on memory, abstract reasoning, calculation, drawing, or writing tasks.[5] If the full test is performed while the patient is confused, a misdiagnosis of dementia can easily be made inadvertently. Because the changes in the brain are physiologic rather than structural, the patient's level of functioning should eventually return to premorbid levels.

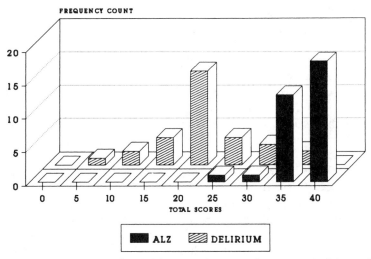

FIGURE 2 – 1. Distribution of total delirium scale scores of patients with Alzheimer's disease versus patients with delirium. In a series of patients, patients with delirium scored an average of 20 points, whereas age-matched patients with Alzheimer's disease averaged 35.

However, the confusion is often slow to clear, and definitive mental status testing to evaluate a possible underlying dementia should be postponed accordingly.

Although the acute onset of inattention, agitation, fluctuating levels of alertness, incoherent speech and train of thought, and visual hallucinations is most often due to a medical condition, the differential diagnosis must include various functional psychiatric disorders such as acute schizophrenic episode, severe anxiety or panic state, agitated depression, and mania. Differentiating between the acute organic confusional states and acute severe functional disorders is difficult but is usually done accurately with data provided from the patient's medical and psychiatric history, the medical examination, and some aspects of the mental status examination. Alterations in the level of consciousness are almost invariably associated with organic brain disease. Visual hallucinations are more typically seen in organic brain disease, whereas auditory hallucinations are more common in functional psychoses. Systematized delusions and organized paranoid ideation are infrequent in patients in an acute confusional state. Whenever the etiology is unclear, the psychiatrist, neurologist, and primary physician should work closely together to conduct a full evaluation.

Frontal Lobe Syndrome

Patients with bilateral frontal lobe disease typically do not show dramatic cognitive deficits on formal mental status testing but often demonstrate specific personality changes.[3,17] The most common features of the frontal lobe personality are (1) apathy, demonstrated both during the examination and toward work and family; (2) euphoria, with a tendency toward jocularity; (3) short-lived irritability; and (4) social inappropriateness.[8]

Some patients with frontal lobe disease are predominantly apathetic, showing little interest in any aspect of their environment.[29] In such patients, the apathy is sometimes misconstrued as depression, a common error by both family and medical personnel. Although these patients are primarily apathetic, they may briefly become very irritable and argumentative when sufficiently stressed.

Conversely, other patients are primarily loud, jocular, inappropriately intrusive, or socially aggressive. Because of their outgoing behavior, these patients may give the initial impression of interest and productivity. However, this emotional disinhibition and euphoria does not result in constructive activity. In general, patients with frontal damage have lost both their interest in their environment and their productive social drive. Such patients often fail to maintain job performance, normal family relations, or even personal cleanliness. Because the frontal lobes are the areas of the brain in which reason and emotion interact,[20] bilateral damage may leave the individual with apathy, unchecked emotions, and an intellect that lacks social and emotional guidance. Other deficits that have been described in patients with frontal lobe damage are higher-order cognitive problems, inattention, memory disorders, and executive motor deficits.[17]

Behavioral features of the frontal lobe syndrome vary from patient to patient, depending partly on the locus of the lesion. Basal-orbital lesions more frequently result in disinhibited, euphoric behavior, with a lack of concern and quick irritability. In contrast, lesions involving the dorsolateral convexities tend to produce apathy, reduced drive, depressed mentation, and impaired planning.[28] See Damasio and Anderson for an excellent comprehensive review of this topic.[7]

The following are two clinical examples of patients with frontal lobe syndromes.

Mrs. L, a 58-year-old housewife, was brought to the hospital by her daughter, who reported that for the past year her mother had shown a decreased interest in caring for her house and personal needs. The patient lived alone in a rural area with few neighbors. The daughter, during an infrequent visit, had noticed a change in her mother's behavior; she showed a lack of interest in conversation and had an unkempt appearance, with a lack of concern about family affairs and total neglect of personal and household cleanliness. Neighbors had noticed that the patient had stopped attending church, did very little shopping, and no longer made social visits. On examination at hospital admission, Mrs. L was awake but markedly apathetic. She offered no spontaneous conversation and answered all questions with only single-word responses. She walked with a slow, shuffling gait and had several episodes of incontinence. Neurodiagnostic evaluation (computed tomography [CT] scan) demonstrated a large frontal cyst. Surgical exploration with drainage produced a marked behavior reversal. Within 2 weeks, the patient was walking well, was conversing spontaneously, and was no longer apathetic or incontinent. Mrs. L represented the primarily apathetic variation of the frontal lobe syndrome.

The next case demonstrates the disinhibition, social inappropriateness, and jocularity that may be associated with the underlying apathy in some patients with this syndrome.

Mr. N was 65 years old when his wife brought him to the hospital. Her chief complaint was that her husband's mind was deranged. She stated that her husband had always been a great joker, but had used proper social restraint until about 4 or 5 years ago, when he had begun to show excessive candor in his remarks to friends and acquaintances. His usual outgoing personality gave way to flippancy and arrogance. His prior restraint was decreased, and he approached each social situation with an almost aggressive egotism, with much showing off and boasting. Over the past years, he had lost regard for his personal cleanliness, bathing and shaving only at his wife's behest. His wife also reported that his memory had started to fail and that he confabulated on occasion. At one point, she had bought a new lawn mower and brought it home with the handle disassembled. She had asked him to put the handle together and to put it on the mower; he had been totally unable to do so.

Later in the course of his disease, Mr. N became quite agitated and paranoid. He wandered around the neighborhood and often told strangers fantastic tales, the most recent being that he "was an undercover agent for the FBI." His judgment in other matters also deteriorated. The last time he drove the car, he went through a stop sign and joked about it with his wife. These latest events prompted his referral to the hospital.

Examination revealed an inattentive, restless, socially inappropriate man who was physically unkempt with uncombed hair, uncut fingernails and toenails, and messy clothes. He exhibited some paranoia, asking if his medicine (Thorazine) was some sort of poison. Several times during the examination he attempted to leave the room and was obviously agitated. His thought processes were extremely concrete, and he performed poorly on virtually all aspects of the mental status examination.

During the hospital period, he became quite upset and irritable, especially at night, and was somewhat aggressive with several nurses. The CT scan revealed frontotemporal atrophy with greatly enlarged frontal horns and widened sulci. The presumptive clinical diagnosis in this case was Pick's disease. He died several years later, and the autopsy verified the diagnosis.

If the behavioral manifestations of the frontal lobe syndrome are present, certain neurologic diseases should be considered in the differential diagnosis: (1) tumors—subfrontal meningiomas, pituitary adenomas, or primary brain tumors; (2) head trauma with frontal contusions; (3) Pick's disease; (4) general paresis; (5) communicating hydrocephalus; (6) Huntington's disease; and (7) AIDS. Any patient with extensive cortical disease (e.g., late Alzheimer's disease, multiple cortical infarcts, or traumatic or postinfectious encephalopathy) exhibits some of the behavior changes seen in patients with frontal lobe disease. However, such patients also show evidence of severe cognitive dysfunction and other indications of pathologic involvement of other brain areas. Interestingly, after mild to moderate closed head injury with frontal lobe contusion, the subsequent behavioral change in certain patients is seen by family members as positive. During the past several years we have seen a number of young adult patients (usually, but not always, male) whose parents and spouses describe "improvements" in mood, reaction to environmental stress, and interactional style after head injury. Unfortunately, the opposite reaction is far more likely.

Disease of the frontal lobes may be difficult to evaluate clinically because of the relative absence of clear-cut cognitive changes associated with lesions in this region.[3,30] However, some clinical tests, primarily "go—don't go" and alternating motor sequencing tasks, can be used to assess frontal lobe function. Luria[19] and others have shown that patients with extensive frontal lobe disease have an impaired ability to perform these tasks.

Alternating Sequences—Visual Pattern Completion Test

DIRECTIONS: Present the patient with the visual patterns from Figure 2–2 on individual sheets of white paper. Tell the patient to reproduce the stimulus figure and then to continue the alternating sequence. If necessary, give additional elaboration of the directions to ensure that the patient understands the nature of the test. Do not correct any errors or provide additional cues after the patient begins the task.

SCORING: Patients with intact motor and sensory systems should be able to complete these sequences without error. A loss of the sequence or perseveration in the reproduction of sequences suggests a loss of the ability to move from one motor movement to another and an inability to shift sets efficiently. Examples of common errors are shown in Figure 2–3.

Alternating Motor Patterns Test

DIRECTIONS: This test consists of a series of changes in hand position. They have been adapted from Luria[19] and are described in greater detail in that source.

1. Fist-Palm-Side Test: Tell the patient to hit the top of the desk repeatedly, first with a fist, then with an open palm, and then with the side of the hand. Demonstrate the task once, and then tell the patient to

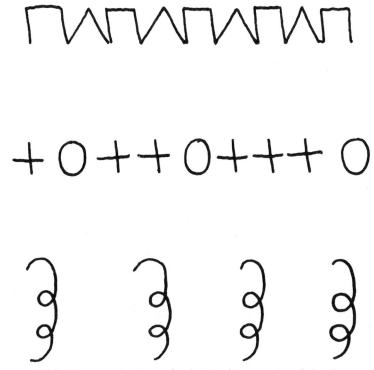

FIGURE 2-2. Test items for the Visual Pattern Completion Test.

perform the task until told to stop. Performance for 15 to 20 seconds should suffice to assess the adequacy of these alternating movements.

2. Fist-Ring Test: Instruct the patient to extend his or her arm several times, first with the hand in a fist, and then with the thumb and forefinger opposed to form a ring. Demonstrate the action, and then tell the patient to perform the action. With successive extensions of the arm, the patient alternates between these two positions.

3. Reciprocal Coordination Test: This alternation test uses both hands. Initially the patient places both hands on the desk, one in a fist and one with the fingers extended palm down. Tell the patient to alternate the position of the two hands rapidly (simultaneously extending the fingers of one hand while making a fist with the other). Demonstrate the task.

SCORING: Normal individuals should have no difficulty in easily mastering these alternating sequences after one or two attempts.[19] Therefore, any appreciable disruption of the smooth performance of these tasks indicates dysfunction of the premotor areas of the cerebral cortex.

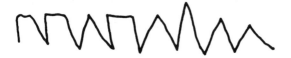

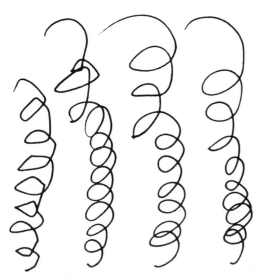

FIGURE 2-3. Common errors in the Visual Pattern Completion Test.

Denial and Neglect

In some patients, a brain lesion may produce a striking degree of **denial of illness**. The following case is an excellent example:

> A surgeon was finishing an operation when his assistant noticed that the surgeon's left arm had suddenly become weak and his speech slurred. The surgeon was immediately put on a stretcher and was brought to the intensive care unit, where one of us saw him within minutes. The patient's arm and face were still weak, but, when asked, he replied, "It is OK." When his weakness was specifically pointed out to him, his comment was, "I really don't recognize any weakness."

This degree of denial seems to result not from a strengthening of normal psychologic defense mechanisms but rather from a more basic and unusual organic behavior change. Clinically the spectrum of denial and neglect syndromes ranges from explicit denial of illness (e.g., the foregoing example), as the most severe behavioral abnormality, to a mild inability to recognize stimulation on one side of the body during bilateral simultaneous stimulation (inattention or extinction). The patient with gross denial may deny total cortical blindness (Anton's syndrome) or a severe hemiparesis (anosognosia).

In many patients with denial, the denial is more implicit than explicit. For example, when asked about the illness, the patient may not actively deny that he or she is ill but may say that he or she is in the hospital for tests to evaluate mild joint pain or some similar benign condition, when in fact they have metastatic cancer. Some patients state that they are not really in a hospital at all, but rather in a rest facility or hotel (reduplication of place or paramnesia). Such patients often make elaborate excuses of fatigue when asked to perform with the paralyzed limb (confabulation) and on occasion will even claim that the weak arm is not theirs at all (reduplication of body parts). The surgeon mentioned earlier, for instance, claimed the next day that he "had some arthritis" in his left arm and that was the reason for his not moving it.

Hemiplegic patients who deny weakness are a great problem in rehabilitation because they are overtly unaware of their weakness and tend to fall repeatedly. One of our patients tried to walk to the bathroom on the first day after his right hemisphere stroke and fell, fracturing his left clavicle.

Some patients do not demonstrate frank denial but do have a dramatic **neglect** of one side of the body. They may shave only one side of the face, use only one sleeve of their robe, and fail to use one side of the body, even though paralysis is not present. These patients also neglect one half of the extrapersonal environment, even in the absence of a visual field defect. For example, patients may fail to respond to a visitor who approaches them from their involved side. Patients may also show neglect on drawing tasks, examples of which are shown in Figure 2–4.

The most subtle form of neglect is an inattention to one side of the body

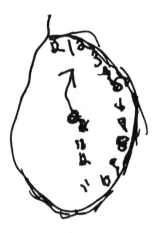

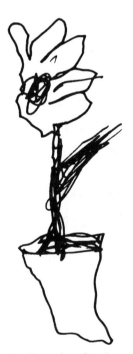

FIGURE 2–4. Examples of neglect on the drawing test.

when both sides are simultaneously stimulated. This tendency to suppress or to extinguish the stimuli on the involved side is discussed in Chapter 4.

The type of lesion that most frequently causes the denial and neglect syndromes is a nondominant hemisphere lesion, usually vascular in etiology.[6] A specific lesion locus within the nondominant hemisphere has not yet been established; subcortical as well as cortical structures may be involved. Gross explicit denial is an uncommon behavioral finding that is most often seen during the acute stages after a vascular accident and is often associated with a degree of confusion. Significant unilateral neglect is also rather uncommon but may be seen as a chronic effect of parietal lesions, predominantly in the nondominant hemisphere. (Patients with frontal lobe disease may also demonstrate denial.) The actual neuropsychologic and neurophysiologic mechanisms underlying these syndromes are not completely understood. For a review of this problem, see references 9, 10, 32, and 33.

Apathy versus Depression or Dysthymia

Apathy, lack of interest in the environment, and psychomotor slowing (psychomotor retardation) are frequently observed in patients with psychiatric depressive illness. However, apathy is but a single symptom and, in isolation, never justifies the diagnosis of depression. Essentially identical symptoms are also characteristic of various organic brain diseases, including frontal lobe lesions, subcortical dementias (e.g., AIDS-related dementia) and other types of dementia, and lesions in the nondominant hemisphere. Because of the critical difference in treatment of depression and of these organic brain diseases, *the importance of differentiating apathy of organic etiology from functional depression cannot be overemphasized.*

Criteria for Diagnosing Depressive Disorders

For the purposes of this book, **depression** refers to a generic affective disorder that consists of several relatively distinct subdisorders and many different symptoms. Within this context, depression includes *major depressive disorder* (*single episode* and *recurrent*), *depressive disorder not otherwise specified*, and *dysthymic disorder*. The diagnostic criteria listed here, adapted from *DSM-IV*, are useful in establishing a diagnosis of one of these disorders of depression, which include but are not totally restricted to the following:

1. Major Depressive Disorder, Single Episode
   By definition, this disorder is time-limited and is of sufficient magnitude to be distinguished from apathy if a careful history is taken.
   A. Presence of a single major depressive episode
      (1) Five or more of the following symptoms are present during the same 2-week period, representing a change from previous functioning:

(a) Depressed mood most of the day, nearly every day
(b) Markedly diminished interest or pleasure in all or most activities
(c) Significant unplanned weight gain or loss
(d) Insomnia or hypersomnia
(e) Psychomotor agitation or retardation
(f) Fatigue or loss of energy
(g) Feelings of worthlessness or excessive guilt
(h) Diminished ability to think or concentrate, or indecisiveness
(i) Recurrent thoughts of death or suicidal ideation

(2) The symptoms do not meet the criteria for any other mood disorder.
(3) The symptoms cause significant distress or impairment of functioning.
(4) The symptoms are not due to the direct effect of a chemical substance (drugs) or a general medical condition.
(5) The symptoms cannot be accounted for by a grief reaction, persist for more than 2 months, or are characterized by marked functional impairment, morbid preoccupation with worthlessness, suicidal ideation, psychotic symptoms, or psychomotor retardation.

B. The major depressive disorder is not caused by, or superimposed on, any other major psychiatric disorder.
C. The patient has never had any type of elevated mood disorder (e.g., mania).

2. Major Depressive Disorder, Recurrent
Behavioral changes associated with this disorder are of sufficient magnitude and duration to warrant careful differentiation from organic apathy in any patient presenting with either "depressive" or "apathetic" symptoms.
A. Two or more major depressive episodes, as defined in the previous section, are present.
B. The episodes are not caused by, or superimposed on, any other type of psychotic disorder (e.g., schizophrenia).

3. Depressive Disorder Not Otherwise Specified
In general, these affective disorders do reach a magnitude that would result in a behavioral change that could be confused with organic apathy. This category includes examples of affective disorders with depressive features that do not meet the criteria for any other depressive disorder:
A. Premenstrual mood disorder
B. Minor depressive disorder
C. Recurrent periods of brief depression
D. Depression following a period of active psychosis

   E. Situations in which the clinician concludes that a depressive dis-
      order is present but cannot determine whether it is primary, due
      to a general medical condition, or substance-induced
4. Dysthymic Disorder
   A. Depressed mood for most of the day, more days than not, for 2
      years.
   B. The presence, while depressed, of two or more of the following:
      (1) Poor appetite or overeating
      (2) Insomnia or hypersomnia
      (3) Low energy or fatigue
      (4) Low self-esteem
      (5) Poor concentration or difficulty making decisions
      (6) Feelings of hopelessness
   C. During the 2-year period, the person has not been without symp-
      toms for more than 2 months at a time.
   D. No major depressive disorder has been present during the 2-year
      period.
   E. The patient has never had a period of abnormally elevated mood.
   F. The disturbance does not occur exclusively during the course of a
      chronic psychotic disorder.
   G. The symptoms are not due to the direct physiologic effects of a
      substance (e.g., drugs) or to a general medical condition (e.g.,
      hypothyroidism).

Differentiating between Depression and Dementia

Before even considering a diagnosis of neurologic disease, the clinician should
carefully evaluate any patient presenting with apathy of nonacute onset as an
initial symptom for the possible presence of a primary depressive disorder.
One of the most common diagnostic dilemmas in this regard is the differentiation between depression and early dementia. Because both conditions
are relatively common in the older population and, more importantly, share
many common features, a misdiagnosis of one for the other is all too easily
made. The significance of such an error is obvious. To tell a depressed individual that he or she is demented is a devastating mistake but one that is no
less significant than overlooking a frontal meningioma while treating the patient for depression.

   One can easily see why diagnoses can become confused: patients with
either condition can present with subjective or repeated complaints of apathy,
loss of interest in work and pleasurable activities, preoccupation with minor
or imagined physical complaints, difficulty concentrating, memory problems,
and a general inability to keep up with the demands of everyday life.

   The problem is further compounded in the elderly. These patients, when depressed, do not always manifest an obviously depressive mood as dramatically as do younger patients. The elderly depressive patient also typically demonstrates fewer crying spells, less expressed sadness, less suicidal ideation (although there is no less threat of actual suicide), less expressed guilt, and less self-deprecation.[24] The elderly depressive patient may also show subtle cognitive deficits on formal mental status testing. No specific pattern of deficits is seen, and the deficits are usually mild.[4] Mild problems with concentration, memory, and arithmetic are common; drawings may contain a paucity of details. In general, performance may be impaired on any task that requires the marshaling of significant mental energy.

Because of the similarity of clinical presentation, it is not surprising that many elderly depressive patients are initially diagnosed as having a dementia.[21] **Pseudodementia**, or dementia of depression, refers to patients giving the initial diagnostic impression of a dementia, but whose symptoms, on careful evaluation and follow-up, prove to be secondary to depression or another emotional disorder and improve with appropriate treatment.[14,23]

The differentiation of true early dementia from pseudodementia is not always easy. Wells[34] has tabulated the major features that can help make this distinction.

Differential Features of Pseudodementia and Dementia

	Pseudodementia	*Dementia*
Clinical course and history	Onset fairly well demarcated	Onset indistinct
	History short	History quite long before consultation
	Rapidly progressive	Early deficits that often go unnoticed
	History of previous psychiatric difficulty or recent life crisis	Uncommon occurrence of previous psychiatric problems or emotional crisis
Clinical behavior	Detailed, elaborate complaints of cognitive dysfunction	Little complaint of cognitive loss
	Little effort expended on examination items	Struggles with cognitive tasks
	Affective change often present	Usually apathetic with shallow emotions
	Behavior does not reflect cognitive loss	Behavior compatible with cognitive loss
	Nocturnal exacerbation rare	Nocturnal accentuation of dysfunction common
Examination findings	Frequently answers "I don't know" before even trying	Usually tries items
	Inconsistent memory loss for both recent and remote items	Memory loss for recent items worse than for remote items
	May have particular memory gaps	No specific memory gaps exist
	Generally inconsistent performance	Rather consistently impaired performance

In our experience, if the examiner takes sufficient time and encourages optimum performance from the patient, the depressed patient with complaints of memory loss will show normal or near-normal performance that is far better than would be expected from the nature and severity of the complaints. In some significantly depressed patients, the mental status examination seems to verify the initial impression of dementia, hence the term "pseudodementia." Because the cognitive examination actually demonstrates impairment that seems organic and is probably caused by chemical (neurotransmitter) abnormalities, the terms "depressive dementia" and "dementia of depression" have been used in preference to "pseudodementia."

The syndrome of pseudodementia is most commonly seen in the elderly depressed patient, but somatoform disorders, manic episodes, high-level anxiety, and any psychotic disorder can produce a picture of dementia on mental status examination. In these cases, it is the inattention, racing thoughts, and confused thinking that preclude adequate performance on the examination. A number of patients with mild closed head injury and major emotional adjustment disorders may also present clinically and on screening examinations with cognitive performance resembling mild dementia because of reduced cognitive efficiency. Treating a patient with pseudodementia is rewarding because, with appropriate treatment, the patient's mental status will revert to normal, premorbid levels.

SUMMARY

Organic brain lesions may cause a multiplicity of behavioral syndromes, some of which are characteristic of specific clinical conditions. The examiner must be prepared to make a systematic evaluation of the patient's behavior and be able to recognize these major neurobehavioral syndromes. The patient's history and behavior provide essential information and serve as a framework for the interpretation of data subsequently obtained from the mental status examination.

REFERENCES

1. American Psychiatric Association: Diagnostic and Statistical Manual of Mental Disorders, ed 4 (DSM-IV). American Psychiatric Association, Washington, DC, 1994.
2. Anderson, NC and Black, DW: Introductory Textbook of Psychiatry. American Psychiatric Press, Washington, DC, 1995.
3. Black, FW: Cognitive deficits in patients with unilateral war-related frontal lobe lesions. J Clin Psychol 32:307, 1976.
4. Caine, ED: Pseudodementia: Current concepts and future directions. Arch Gen Psychiatry 38:1359, 1981.
5. Chédru, F and Geschwind, N: Writing disturbances in acute confusional states. Neuropsychologia 10:343, 1972.
6. Critchley, M: The Parietal Lobes. Edward Arnold & Co., London, 1953.
7. Damasio, AR and Anderson, SW: The frontal lobes: In Heilman, KM and Valenstein, E (eds): Clinical Neuropsychology. Oxford University Press, New York, 1993, pp 409–460.

8. Hécaen, H and Albert, ML: Disorders of mental functioning related to frontal lobe pathology. In Benson, DF and Blumer, D (eds): Psychiatric Aspects of Neurologic Disease. Grune & Stratton, New York, 1975, pp 137–149.

9. Heilman, KM, et al: Localization of lesions in neglect. In Kertesz, A (ed): Localization in Neuropsychology. Academic Press, New York, 1983, pp 471–492.

10. Heilman, KM, Watson, RT, and Valenstein, E: Neglect and related disorders. In Heilman, KM and Valenstein, E (eds): Clinical Neuropsychology, ed 3. Oxford University Press, New York, 1993, pp. 279–336.

11. Inouye, SK and Charpentier, PA: Precipitating factors for delirium in hospitalized elderly persons. JAMA 275:852–857, 1996.

12. Janowsky, DS: Pseudodementia in the elderly: Differential diagnosis and treatment. J Clin Psychiatry 43:19, 1982.

13. Kaplan, HI and Sadock, BJ: Modern Synopsis of Comprehensive Textbook of Psychiatry. Williams & Wilkins, Baltimore, 1988.

14. Kiloh, LG: Pseudo-dementia. Acta Psychiatr Scand 37:336, 1961.

15. Lerner, AJ, Hedera, P, Koss, E, et al: Delirium in Alzheimer disease. Alzheimer Dis Assoc Disord 11:16–20, 1997.

16. Levenson, AJ (ed): Neuropsychiatric Side-Effects of Drugs in the Elderly. Raven Press, New York, 1979.

17. Levin, HS, Eisenberg, HM, and Benton, AL (eds): Frontal Lobe Function and Dysfunction. Oxford University Press, New York, 1991.

18. Lishman, WA: Organic Psychiatry: The Psychological Consequences of Cerebral Disorders. Blackwell Science, London, 1998.

19. Luria, AR: Traumatic Aphasia. Moulton & Co, The Hague, Netherlands, 1970.

20. Nauta, WJH: The problem of the frontal lobe: A reinterpretation. J Psychiatr Res 8:167, 1971.

21. Nott, PN and Fleminger, JJ: Presenile dementia: The difficulties of early diagnosis. Acta Psychiatr Scand 51:210, 1975.

22. Pompei, P, Foreman, M, Cassel, CK, et al: Detecting delirium among hospitalized older patients. Arch Intern Med 155:301–307, 1995.

23. Post, F: Dementia, depression and pseudo-dementia. In Benson, DF and Blumer, D (eds): Psychiatric Aspects of Neurologic Disease. Grune & Stratton, New York, 1975, pp 99–120.

24. Reese, WL, Lipsedge, M and Ball, C (eds): Textbook of Psychiatry. Oxford University Press, New York, 1997.

25. Strauss, ED: The psychiatric interview, history, and mental status examination. In Kaplan, HI and Sadock, BJ (eds): Comprehensive Textbook of Psychiatry. Williams & Wilkins, Baltimore, 1995, pp 521–531.

26. Strub, RL: Acute confusional state. In Benson, DF and Blumer, D (eds): Psychiatric Aspects of Neurologic Disease, Vol II. Grune & Stratton, New York, 1982, pp 1–21.

27. Strub, RL: Mental disorders in brain disease. In Frederiks, JAM (ed): Handbook of Clinical Neurology, Vol 2 (46), Neurobehavioral Disorders. Elsevier Science Publishers, Amsterdam, 1985, pp 413–441.

28. Stuss, DT and Benson, DF: Frontal lobe lesions and behavior. In Kertesz, A (ed): Localization in Neuropsychology. Academic Press, New York, 1983, pp 429–454.

29. Stuss, DT and Benson, DF: Neuropsychological studies of the frontal lobes. Psychol Bull 95:3, 1984.

30. Teuber, HL: The riddle of frontal lobe function in man. In Warren, J and Alert, K (eds): The Frontal Granular Cortex and Behavior. McGraw-Hill, New York, 1964, pp 410–440.

31. Trzepacz, PT and Baker, RW: The Psychiatric Mental Status Examination. Oxford University Press, New York, 1993.

32. Weinstein, EA and Friedland, RP: Hemi-inattention and Hemispheric Specialization. Advances in Neurology, Vol 18. Raven Press, New York, 1977.

33. Weinstein, EA and Kahn, RL: Denial of illness. Charles C Thomas, Springfield, IL, 1955.

34. Wells, CE: Pseudodementia. Am J Psychiatry 136:895, 1979.

LEVELS OF CONSCIOUSNESS

The initial step in administering a formal mental status examination is to determine the patient's level of consciousness. This basic brain function determines the patient's ability to relate both to self and to the environment. Any disturbance of this elementary function almost invariably affects the higher-level mental processes that constitute the major portion of the mental status examination. An alteration in level of consciousness is an important indicator of brain dysfunction and is usually caused either by primary neurologic disease or systemic medical illness.

The term **consciousness** is multifaceted; in testing consciousness, it is important to distinguish between the content of consciousness and basic arousal.[10] **Content** refers to higher cognitive and emotional functioning, whereas **arousal** refers to the activation of the cortex from the ascending activating system (brain stem reticular formation and the diffuse thalamic projection system). Content and arousal can vary independently, and the final level of consciousness represents a dynamic balance between cortical and ascending activating systems. This chapter deals with the clinical aspects of basic arousal.

TERMINOLOGY AND EVALUATION

Many general terms are used to describe the basic levels of consciousness, which represent points on a continuum from full alertness to deep coma. Most clinicians distinguish five principal levels: (1) alertness, (2) lethargy or somnolence, (3) obtundation, (4) stupor or semicoma, and (5) coma.

Alertness implies that the patient is awake and fully aware of normal external and internal stimuli. Barring paralysis, the patient can respond appropriately to any normal stimulus. The alert patient is able to interact in a meaningful way with the examiner. In cases of total paralysis, eye contact or eye movement may be adequate to establish this interaction. Because there are unusual comalike states in which alertness is simulated, we feel that an observation of alertness should be predicated on the clinician's impression that meaningful interpersonal interaction is taking place. Alertness per se does not imply the inherent capacity to focus attention, a topic to be discussed in detail in Chapter 4.

Lethargy, or somnolence, is a state in which the patient is not fully alert and tends to drift off to sleep when not actively stimulated. In such patients, spontaneous movements are decreased and awareness is limited. When aroused, these patients are usually unable to pay close attention to the examiner; their eyes are open and directed toward the examiner, yet they appear dull and without animation. In conversation, the lethargic patient often loses the train of thought and wanders from topic to topic. It is difficult to assess memory, calculations, and abstract thinking with validity in these patients because of their inattention and wandering thought processes. If a lethargic patient takes a full mental status examination, impaired performance must be interpreted with caution.

Obtundation is a transitional state between lethargy and stupor. The obtunded patient is difficult to arouse and, when aroused, is confusional. Usually, constant stimulation is required to elicit even marginal cooperation from the patient. Meaningful mental status testing is usually futile. The obtunded patient is, by our definition, in an acute confusional state or quiet delirium.

Stupor and **semicoma** are used to describe patients who respond only to persistent and vigorous stimulation. The stuporous patient does not rouse spontaneously and, when aroused by the examiner, can only groan or mumble and move restlessly in the bed. In such a patient, there is extensive brain dysfunction; because of the markedly reduced level of consciousness, no meaningful assessment of the content of mental functioning is possible.

Coma is traditionally applied to those patients who are completely unarousable and remain with their eyes closed. In coma, the patient responds neither to external stimulation nor spontaneously to internal stimulation. If coma is thus defined as a state in which no evidence of behavioral response to stimulation is present, the term can serve as an absolute end point on the scale of consciousness or arousability. Some clinicians make a distinction between light coma and deep coma. In light coma, the patient may demonstrate reflex (e.g., decorticate or decerebrate) movements but no meaningful or purposeful movements, whereas in deep coma, no motor response is seen at all. Stupor and coma are not discussed further here; the interested reader is referred to Plum and Posner;[10] Young, Ropper, and Bolton;[13] and Fisher[3] for extensive discussions of these states.

Each of the aforementioned terms is qualitative and encompasses a wide range of possible points on the continuum of consciousness. Such terms lack the objectivity and reliability that can be achieved with a less subjective assessment scheme. We suggest amending any qualitative term such as "lethargy" with a series of short statements that describe both the level of stimulus

TABLE 3 – 1. Patient's Responses to Stimulation

	Level of Consciousness	Stimulus Necessary to Rouse Patient	Movement	Vocalization	Eye Opening	Comments
8 PM	Lethargy	Loud voice	Moved all limbs; got up on elbow	Mumbled something about being tired	Yes, with eye contact	Odor of alcohol on breath
12 AM	Lethargy	Loud voice plus gentle shaking	Moved all limbs; no attempt to rise	Incoherent mumbling	Yes, but with no sustained eye contact	Questionable Babinski's sign
4 AM	Stupor	Loud voice plus vigorous shaking	Slight movement of all extremities, but right arm not moving well	Groans	Attempted to open eyes to command	Left pupil larger than right, not as reactive; now positive Babinski's sign on right

necessary to arouse the patient, the actual behavioral response elicited, and what the patient does when the stimulation ceases.

First, *the intensity of stimulation needed to arouse the patient* should be indicated: (1) calling the patient's name in a normal conversational tone, (2) calling in a loud voice, (3) light touch on the arm, (4) vigorous shaking of the patient's shoulder, or (5) painful stimulation. Second, the *patient's highest-level responses* should be described: (1) degree and quality of movement, (2) presence and coherence of speech, or (3) presence of eye opening and eye contact with the examiner. Finally, *what the patient does on cessation of stimulation* should be described.

This information can be recorded in a single statement. For example:

- Patient *lethargic*: Patient's name called in a normal tone of voice; patient opened eyes, pulled self part way up in bed, mumbled "Why ya bothering me?" then closed eyes and went back to sleep.
- Patient *obtunded*: Responded to loud shouting with restless movements of all extremities and brief eye opening; speech mumbled and incoherent; when stimulation discontinued, patient returned to sleep.
- Patient *stuporous*: Did not respond to voice but responded to vigorous shaking of shoulder, accompanied by loud calling of patient's name, with groan and aimless movement of left extremities; eyes remained closed.

These types of descriptions provide much more data on the patient's arousability and capacity for interaction than the simple terms "lethargy," "obtundation," or "stupor." It is helpful to make a chart in the progress notes so that a rapid assessment of changing levels of consciousness can be made. Table 3–1 is an example of a patient with head trauma who had a subdural

TABLE 3 – 2. **Glasgow Coma Scale***		
Category of Response	*Response*	*Points*
Eye opening	Spontaneous	4
	To speech	3
	To pain	2
	Nil	1
Best verbal response	Oriented	5
	Confused conversation	4
	Inappropriate words	3
	Incomprehensible	2
	Nil	1
Best motor response	Obeys	6
	Localizes	5
	Withdraws	4
	Abnormal flexion (decorticate)	3
	Extends (decerebrate)	2
	Nil	1

*Adapted from Jennett and Teasdale,[6] p. 78.

TABLE 3 – 3. Glasgow Coma Scale Graph

Patient's Response	Date	12 PM	2 PM	4 PM	6 PM	8 PM	10 PM	12 AM
Eye opening								
Spontaneous								
To speech		•	•					
To pain				•				
None					•	•	•	
Best verbal response								
Oriented								
Confused								
Inappropriate			•	•				
Incomprehensible					•	•	•	
None		•						
Best motor response								
Obeying								
Localizing		•	•					
Withdraws				•				
Flexing					•	•		
Extending							•	
None								
Coma Score		12	11	8	6	6	4	

hematoma. As shifts of nurses and doctors change, subtle changes in the patient's condition are easily appreciated by comparing the notes of previous observers. This system is applicable to any patient whose illness causes a decrease in the level of awareness.

Teasdale and Jennett[6,12] have demonstrated the practicality of this type of reporting system for patients with head injury. They have developed what has become known as the Glasgow Coma, or Responsiveness, Scale. It follows the conceptual scheme described earlier but has the advantage of providing a numeric score to denote the actual level of consciousness. Each level of response in the three response categories (i.e., eye opening, verbal, motor) is given a numeric value. The response is the patient's best response; it does not, however, take into account the level of stimulus required for its elicitation. The scale items and the quantitative ratings for specific responses are presented in Table 3–2. Additionally, the Rancho Los Amigos Scale[4,7] is commonly used to track the patient's level of consciousness and responsiveness to environmental stimuli in rehabilitation settings.

The level of responsiveness can be assessed objectively at regular intervals and plotted as a graph. The time scale can be hourly, daily, or any selected interval. Table 3–3 is an example of such use of the scale.

ANATOMY AND CLINICAL IMPLICATIONS

The basic brain structure responsible for arousal is the ascending activating system. This system originates in the brain stem reticular formation and extends to the cortex via the diffuse or nonspecific thalamic projection system.[9]

A group of specialized reticular neurons in the tegmental portion of the midbrain and upper pons has the specific capacity to activate higher centers. These cells are located in a perimedian portion in the brain stem (reticular formation and locus ceruleus) and receive collateral input from most ascending and descending fiber systems. Stimulation applied to the skin of the hand, for example, will send information to the activating system as well as the sensory nuclei in the thalamus. Reticular stimulation alerts widespread areas of the cortex and subcortex to the fact that an external stimulus is being applied. By this mechanism, the activating system maintains a constant, albeit fluctuating, stimulation of the higher centers. Without this steady input, the cortex cannot function efficiently; thus, the patient cannot think clearly, learn effectively, or relate meaningfully. Any damage or suppression of this system renders the patient difficult to arouse and inefficient in performance. Specific lesions such as infarcts or hemorrhages of the reticular formation lead to total disruption of arousal and, thus, to coma. Pressure on the midbrain from hippocampal or uncal herniation causes a change in the level of consciousness, which starts as lethargy but may progress to coma. Drug intoxication, disturbances in metabolic balance, and sepsis cause alterations in both reticular and cortical functioning. This leads to alterations not only in arousal, but also in the content of consciousness.

If there is damage to the extension of the brain stem reticular system in the thalamus or hypothalamus, the full picture of coma will not result. Such lesions disconnect the reticulocortical and reticulolimbic pathways and cause patients to display various interesting alterations in arousal. Because the brain stem portion of the system is intact, reticular activity innervates the nuclei of the extraocular nerves, and patients can open their eyes and look about. The cortex, however, is not sufficiently stimulated to produce voluntary movement or speech. These patients are in a comalike state.

These unusual comalike states are interesting because of the nature and degree of disturbed awareness. Some authors categorize all such cases as **akinetic mutism** or **persistent vegetative states**, whereas others prefer to separate them into their many subcategories. Regardless of the terminology used, however, the pathology and clinical appearance of each subcategory are relatively distinct. The primary feature of patients with these disorders is the uncanny appearance of awareness. Such patients lie in bed with their eyes open and look about the room. Eye contact with others is variable. Sometimes eye movements seem random, but on other occasions, genuine interpersonal eye contact appears to take place. Other than this somewhat unnerving visual scanning, the patients remain relatively immobile and mute. It is the dichotomy between this apparent visual alertness and the lack of speech and movement that differentiates this group of patients from those in stupor or coma. The critical defining features of this vegetative state, as with coma, are no evidence of awareness of self or the environment and no evidence that the patient can understand or communicate with an examiner.[1]

Regardless of their superficial similarity, each subgroup of the comalike states has its own distinct features; it is often possible to differentiate among the various states clinically and to separate them from a true vegetative state. The term "akinetic mutism" seems best reserved for patients in whom damage is restricted either to the midbrain or subthalamic region or to the septal region.

A midbrain lesion causes a syndrome called **apathetic akinetic mutism**. Patients with this syndrome are difficult to arouse but, once aroused, can move all extremities, mutter a few intelligible words, and look directly at the examiner for a few moments. They then turn away or drift back to sleep. Subtle muscle stretch reflex changes, extensor toe signs, extraocular muscle involvement, and pupillary abnormalities may be seen. Although this condition was originally described in a patient with a third ventricular cyst,[2] the most common cause is occlusion of the small vessels entering the brain stem from the tip of the basilar artery.[11] This lesion interrupts the ascending activating system but not the corticospinal and corticobulbar tracts. Accordingly, the patients can open their eyes and make some movement and sound but are unable to respond fully. Because of the akinetic mute patients' capacity to interact with the environment, they are not in a vegetative state.

Patients with lesions that involve the septal area, anterior hypothalamus, cingulate gyri, or bilateral orbital frontal cortex are also akinetic and mute but appear much more alert. These patients are awake most of the day and have insomnia at night, their eyes remaining open while they are awake. Described as being in a coma vigil, these individuals often have violent behavioral outbursts during arousal (septal rage). This syndrome is seen in those with rupture of anterior communicating artery aneurysms, deep frontal lobe tumors, and anterior cingulate gyrus tumors. Increased leg reflexes, with Babinski's sign from corticospinal tract involvement, difficulty with temperature control from anterior hypothalamic damage, and primitive reflexes (snout and grasp) from mesial frontal lobe damage may be seen. These patients do not have pupillary or extraocular muscle paresis. These neurologic signs, plus the more apparent alertness of these patients, frequently differentiates them clinically from apathetic akinetic mute patients.

Patients with diffuse damage to the cortical mantle from anoxia, hypoglycemia, or circulatory or metabolic embarrassment frequently survive in a state clinically similar to that of coma vigil. Their eyes are open and randomly survey the room. Brain stem reflexes are intact, but bilateral decortication with double hemiplegia and primitive reflexes is present. This condition is called the **apallic state**[8] because of the diffuse damage to the isocortex. Because of the dramatic neurologic deficit, this state should be easily distinguished from the akinetic mute states.

The term "persistent vegetative state" has been used to describe patients surviving severe head injury whose symptoms are clinically similar to those in the apallic state.[5] The brain lesions are widespread at both the cortical and subcortical levels, and neurologic findings differ in each case, depending on the specific loci of the lesions. Because the term "apallic state" has never gained widespread acceptance, "persistent vegetative state" is often used for any patient with widespread brain disease and no ability to interact meaningfully with the environment.

The **locked-in syndrome**[10] is another comalike state that can be differentiated from the foregoing states. In this condition, a lesion (hemorrhage or infarct) in the upper pontine tegmentum interrupts all corticospinal and corticobulbar fibers at the level of the abducens and facial nuclei. Clinically, patients are unable to speak, swallow, smile, or move their limbs. In some cases, lateral gaze is also paralyzed. The entire central nervous system above the level of the lesion is intact, and these patients are literally disconnected from their motor system. These patients are "locked-in" and able to communicate by eye movements only.

Table 3–4 is a composite of the clinical features of each of these comalike

TABLE 3-4. Diagnostic Features of Comalike States

Diagnosis	Level of Consciousness	Voluntary Movement	Speech	Eye Responses	Limb Tone	Reflexes
Akinetic mute (apathetic-midbrain)	Lethargy	Little and infrequent; but when sufficiently stimulated, can move **all** extremities purposefully	With stimulation, can produce normal, short phrases	Open when stimulated; usually good eye contact	Usually normal; sometimes slight increase	Can be normal; occasionally asymmetric with pathologic reflexes
Akinetic mute (coma vigil-septal)	Wakeful, with occasional outbursts; some patients somnolent	Little but purposeful; arms usually move much better than legs	Little; can occasionally produce normal phrases; also can have outbursts of unintelligible utterances	Open during much of the day in most patients; eye contact variable	Often increased in legs	Frequently have increased leg reflexes; Babinski's signs, snout, grasp often present
Apallic state (decorticate)	Awake: no meaningful interaction with environment	No or little purposeful movement; mostly reflex or mass movements	None or occasional grunting	Open, searching, but no real eye contact	Increased in all extremities; extremities often in flexion	Increase in all extremities with pathologic reflexes
Persistent vegetative state	Awake; no interaction with environment	None	None	Open, searching, but no real eye contact	Variable, usually increased; extremities often in flexion	Variable, usually increased with pathologic reflexes
Locked-in syndrome	Awake and alert; able to communicate meaningfully with examiners by eye movement	None or slight, except for eye movement	None	Open, with normal following and good eye contact; some patients have restricted lateral gaze	Increased	Increased in all extremities

37

states. These features plus the clinical history should enable the examiner to differentiate most of these complicated cases.

A final condition that deserves mention in this section is the state of **psychogenic unresponsiveness** (also called hysterical comalike state or somatoform disorder/conversion disorder). This condition constitutes 1% of all patients presenting to a medical emergency room in an unresponsive state.[10] Careful examination reveals normal respiration, heart rate, and blood pressure. Muscle tone is usually decreased, but inconsistent limb tone frequently exists. All bulbar reflexes (doll's eye phenomenon, caloric stimulation, gag, corneal, and pupil) are intact. Muscle stretch reflexes are symmetric. Frequently, the patient will make inconsistent responses, such as blinking on corneal testing before the cornea is touched. Any inconsistent response gives the examiner additional confidence that the patient does not have a medical or neurologically induced coma. Psychogenic unresponsiveness should not be diagnosed too hastily; mistakenly labeling a true coma as psychogenic unresponsiveness is far more serious than the reverse.

All of the conditions discussed earlier represent disturbances of arousal caused by brain lesions or psychiatric illness. *Not all alterations in levels of alertness are pathologic, however.* Sleep, for instance, represents a natural fluctuation in the level of consciousness. Any degree of fatigue or sleepiness can adversely affect performance on mental status testing, even in the absence of an organic lesion. Patients with brain disease continue to have an underlying diurnal sleep-wake cycle that is superimposed on any organic decrease in alertness. It may be difficult to determine the relative effects of sleep and pathologic alterations in the level of consciousness, but the examiner must consider both factors in the evaluation. For example, the patient with head trauma who is difficult to arouse on morning rounds may only be asleep and not suffering from increasing intracranial pressure. In these critical cases, the observed level of awareness is not the only critical factor that determines the necessity for therapeutic intervention. The patient's neurologic status and overall hospital course must also be considered.

SUMMARY

Because consciousness is the most rudimentary of all mental functions, consciousness level must be determined first in any mental status examination. Any alteration in the level of consciousness decreases the efficiency of cortical functioning, and thereby significantly decreases the validity of the subsequent steps in the mental status examination. In the patient with diminished alertness, only the more obvious changes in higher cognitive function can be validly documented.

The ascending activating system controls the arousal aspect of consciousness. Any damage to or dysfunction of this subcortical system alters alertness and thus secondarily affects cortical activity.

REFERENCES

1. American Neurological Association Committee on Ethical Affairs: Persistent vegetative state: Report of the American Neurological Committee on Ethical Affairs. Ann Neurol 33:386–390, 1993.
2. Cairns, H, et al: Akinetic mutism with an epidermoid cyst of the third ventricle. Brain 64:273, 1941.
3. Fisher, CM: The neurological examination of the comatose patient. Acta Neurol Scand (Suppl) 36:1, 1969.
4. Hagan, C: Language disorders in head trauma. In Holland, A (ed): Language Disorders in Adults. College-Hill Press, San Diego, CA, 1984.
5. Jennett, B and Plum, F: Persistent vegetative state after brain damage. Lancet 1:734, 1972.
6. Jennett, B and Teasdale, G: Assessment of impaired consciousness. In Jennett, B and Teasdale, G: Management of Head Injuries. FA Davis, Philadelphia, 1981, pp 77–93.
7. Kay, T and Lezak, MD: The nature of head injury. In Corthell, D (ed): Traumatic Brain Injury and Vocational Rehabilitation. University of Wisconsin, Menomonee, WI, 1990.
8. Kretschmer, E: Das Appalische Syndrom. Z Gesamte Neurol Psychiatr 169:576, 1940.
9. Magoun, H: The Waking Brain. Charles C Thomas, Springfield, IL, 1963.
10. Plum, F and Posner, J: Diagnosis of Stupor and Coma, ed 3. FA Davis, Philadelphia, 1982.
11. Segarra, J and Angelo, J: Anatomical determinants of behavior change. In Benton, A (ed): Behavioral Change in Cerebral Vascular Disease. Harper & Row, New York, 1970, pp 3–14.
12. Teasdale, G and Jennett, B: Assessment of coma and impaired consciousness. Lancet 2:81, 1974.
13. Young, GB, Ropper AH, and Bolton CF (eds): Coma and Impaired Consciousness. McGraw-Hill, New York, 1998.

ATTENTION

After determining the level of consciousness, assessment of attention is the next step in the examination. The patient's ability to sustain attention over time must be established before evaluating the more complex functions such as memory, language, and abstract thinking. It is of no value to ask the patient to remember the details of a story if he or she is repeatedly distracted by internal stimuli or by the nurse passing in the hall, a noise in the next room, or cars in the street. The inattentive and distractible patient cannot efficiently assimilate the information being presented during testing.

Attention is the patient's ability to attend to a specific stimulus without being distracted by extraneous internal or environmental stimuli.[19] This capacity for focusing on a single stimulus contrasts with the concept of alertness or vigilance. The term "vigilance," however, has been used interchangeably with both "sustained attention" (focusing on one stimulus over an extended period of time) and also with the more common concept of "watchfulness" or "alertness."[24] *Vigilance in the sense of alertness refers to a more basic arousal process in which the awake patient can respond to any stimulus appearing in the environment.* The vigilant (alert) but inattentive patient will be attracted to any novel sound, movement, or event occurring in the vicinity; the attentive patient can screen out irrelevant stimuli. Attention presupposes alertness, but alertness does not necessarily imply attentiveness.

Sustained attention (concentration) is the ability to maintain attention to a specific stimulus over an extended period. This capacity to concentrate is very important for performing intellectual endeavors and may be impaired in both medical and emotional disorders. A wide variety of factors have been shown to interfere with attention; the intensity and frequency of the stimulus: environmental stressors (e.g., noise, temperature, complexity of the environment), emotional factors (e.g., anxiety or depression), and to some extent lower IQ.[1] The concept of **inattention (distractibility)** is applied to two distinct clinical situations. The first is when the patient is clinically inattentive or is unable to sustain sufficient attention to succeed in the simple tests of attention discussed subsequently. The second situation is when the patient has specific unilateral inattention (neglect) to stimuli on the side of the body opposite a brain lesion.

EVALUATION

Observation

One of the most valid sources of clinical information regarding the patient's general attentiveness may be obtained by merely observing the patient's behavior and noting any evidence of distractibility or difficulty in attending to the examiner. A subjective rating scale of 0 (highly distractible) to 5 (fully attentive) is useful as a means of quantifying attention over the course of the examination.

History

A patient who is having difficulty concentrating on work or other routine tasks is usually able to tell the examiner about the problem. A simple inquiry as to the patient's ability to concentrate or to sustain attention often provides revealing data.

Digit Repetition

The patient's basic level of attention can be readily assessed by using the **Digit Repetition Test**. Adequate performance on this task ensures that the patient is able to attend to a verbal stimulus and to sustain attention for the period of time required to repeat the digits. In patients with a significant language disorder (aphasia), this task and the "A" Random Letter Test for sustained attention, which follows, cannot be validly applied to assess attention.

DIRECTIONS: Tell the patient: "I am going to say some simple numbers. Listen carefully and when I am finished, say the numbers after me." Present the digits in a normal tone of voice at a rate of one digit per second. Take care not to group digits either in pairs (e.g., 2–6, 5–9) or in sequences that could serve as an aid to repetition (e.g., in telephone number form, 376-8439). Numbers should be presented randomly without natural sequences (e.g., not 2–4–6–8). Begin with a two-number sequence, and continue until the patient fails to repeat all the numbers correctly.

TEST ITEMS

3–7	9–2
7–4–9	1–7–4
8–5–2–7	5–2–9–7
2–9–6–8–3	6–3–8–5–1
5–7–2–9–4–6	2–9–4–7–3–8
8–1–5–9–3–6–2	4–1–9–2–7–5–1
3–9–8–2–5–1–4–7	8–5–3–9–1–6–2–7
7–2–8–5–4–6–7–3–9	2–1–9–7–3–5–8–4–6

SCORING: The patient of average intelligence can accurately repeat five to seven digits without difficulty. In a nonretarded patient without obvious aphasia, inability to repeat more than five digits indicates defective attention. Specific age-related norms for this task are readily available.[10,22,23]

Sustained Attention

A simple test of sustained attention that can be readily administered at the bedside is the "A" Random Letter Test. It consists of a series of random letters among which a target letter appears with greater-than-random frequency. The patient is required to indicate whenever the target letter is spoken by the examiner.

DIRECTIONS: Tell the patient: "I am going to read you a long series of letters. Whenever you hear the letter 'A,' indicate by tapping the desk." Read the following letter list in a normal tone at a rate of one letter per second.

TEST ITEMS

L	T	P	E	A	O	A	I	C	T	D	A	L	A	A
A	N	I	A	B	F	S	A	M	R	Z	E	O	A	D
P	A	K	L	A	U	C	J	T	O	E	A	B	A	A
Z	Y	F	M	U	S	A	H	E	V	A	A	R	A	T

SCORING: Currently, only preliminary standardized norms exist for this test. The average person should complete the task without error ($\bar{x} = 0.2$); a sample of randomly selected brain-damaged patients made an average of 10 errors.[17] Examples of common organic errors are (1) failure to indicate when the target letter has been presented (omission error); (2) indication made when a nontarget letter has been presented (commission error); and (3) failure to stop tapping with the presentation of subsequent nontarget letters (perseveration error).

Another attention test that has been traditionally included in mental status examinations is the Serial Sevens Subtraction Test (e.g., counting backward from 100 by 7s: 100, 93, 86, . . .). Results of studies of performance by normal people suggest that errors on this test may be influenced by intellectual capability, education, calculating ability, or socioeconomic status, rather than indicating a pathologic process.[12,18] Excellent performance indicates adequate attention or mental control, but failure may reflect any of a number of problems, inattention being but one. In general, this test has proved of limited validity.

Unilateral Inattention

Unilateral inattention (suppression or extinction) should be tested during the routine sensory examination by using **double (bilateral) simultaneous stimulation**.

DIRECTIONS: Double simultaneous stimulation is tested in all major sensory modalities. In tactile testing, corresponding points on both sides of the body are touched simultaneously with equal intensity. Visual testing is done by having the patient face the examiner and fix his or her gaze at a point on the examiner's face. The examiner then wiggles a finger in right and left peripheral fields. Auditory testing is carried out by having the examiner stand behind the patient and provide a stimulus of equal intensity to each ear.

Before undertaking bilateral simultaneous stimulation, the examiner must ensure that basic sensation for each modality is intact bilaterally. If one side is inferior on unilateral testing, defects found during simultaneous testing would not necessarily reflect inattention.

Extinction is present when the patient suppresses the stimuli from one side of the body. Extinction may occur in all modalities (polymodal neglect) or may be restricted to a single modality. When extinction is elicited, the degree of inattention can be assessed by increasing the magnitude of the stimulus on the inattentive side.

When the double simultaneous stimulation includes one proximal and one distal stimulus, the distal stimulus tends to be neglected or extinguished.[4] This is particularly true when the proximal stimulus is the face and the distal one the hand. Normal adults under 65 often extinguish the hand stimulus on the first trial but usually begin to identify both stimuli after several trials. Patients with organic brain syndromes rarely recognize the hand stimulus even after as many as 10 trials. This test (Face-Hand Test)[2] is a very useful simple test for organic disease. Some normal elderly individuals will also extinguish the hand stimulus; therefore, the test must be interpreted with caution in patients over 65.

ANATOMY AND CLINICAL IMPLICATIONS

The basic anatomic structures responsible for maintaining an alert state are the brain stem reticular activating system and the diffuse thalamic projection system (the diencephalic extension of the reticular formation).[13]

The mechanism by which this ascending activation is focused and extraneous stimuli are screened out is less certain. Cortical and limbic stimulation can definitely influence the ascending system, so it is probable that attention results from a balance among ascending (reticulocortical) activation, ascending inhibition, and cortical (corticoreticular) modulation.[13] Selectively focusing attention requires a widespread network of cortical neurons, particularly the prefrontal including the posterior cingulate gyrus inferior parietal cortex and medial temporal/occipital cortices.[15] The importance of cortical influence in focusing attention is demonstrated in the experience of every student. Concentration while studying frequently requires conscious voluntary effort that is cortical in origin. The limbic system is also an integral part of the attention process; limbic input adds emotional importance to the object of attention. A child who watches a cartoon is stimulated to pay attention by the pleasure and excitement generated by the spectacle. The student who is studying for a test is aided in the need to concentrate by a fear of failure or a drive to succeed. These limbic influences are important and may be the critical factor that facilitates the screening out of extraneous stimuli. The principal stimulus is of greater emotional value than the incidental events in the environment, and therefore it attracts greater attention.

Because attention represents a complex interaction of limbic, neocortical, and ascending activating functions, *many areas of the brain exist in which damage can disrupt the ability to attend.* Damage to the ascending activating system itself usually causes alterations in the level of consciousness. In such patients, alterations in attention are directly related to the more basic deficit in alertness. Inattention caused by lesions in the midbrain activating system is clinically rare, although a rather profound unilateral inattention has been experimentally produced in monkeys with lesions in the midbrain.[20] Inattention has also been observed clinically in patients with lesions of the thalamus,[21] the posterior internal capsule,[5] and other subcortical structures.[14]

Some of the patients who survived the encephalitis epidemic of 1918 to 1921, which was associated with Economo's disease, were left with lesions in the ascending inhibitory portion of the reticular substance of the pons and medulla. These patients developed a behavior pattern characterized by hyperactivity and distractibility, which was called "organic driveness."[11] This state is clinically similar to that seen in some children with Attention-Deficit/Hyperactivity Disorder (ADHD).

Probably the most common cause of decreased attention and vigilance in a hospital population is diffuse brain dysfunction (delirium). This dysfunction, in which all cells in the central nervous system are affected, is usually caused by metabolic disturbance, drug intoxication, postsurgical states, or systemic infection. Another common cause of inattention is extensive bilateral cortical damage of any etiology (e.g., atrophy, multiple infarcts, encephalitis, or head trauma). In patients with advanced Alzheimer's dementia, for example, new stimuli in the vicinity may quickly draw their attention and they then become "stimulus bound." The cortical role in focusing and maintaining attention is very well demonstrated in these patients.

Patients with bilateral lesions of the frontal lobes or the limbic system (e.g., Korsakoff's syndrome) have a type of inattention that is characterized by indifference and perseveration. Clinically, they are apathetic toward their surroundings and are not particularly interested in test items per se. Such patients usually perform well on the digit repetition task but cannot complete the "A" Random Letter Test accurately. These patients often fail to recognize an "A" at the end of a long sequence (e.g., U C J T O E A) because their attention has wandered. Patients with a frontal lobe lesion also have great difficulty shifting from one pattern of response to another, resulting in perseveration. This perseveration is commonly seen both behaviorally and on the "A" Random Letter Test. For example, the series E V A A R A T may be failed by an individual with perseveration in the following way (italic letters indicate the patient's taps): E V *A A* R A *T*.

Right hemisphere lesions have a stronger effect on attention than do left-sided lesions. Denial, unilateral neglect, and extinction on double simultaneous stimulation occur more frequently and are more prominent in patients with right hemisphere lesions.[2,6,7,16] The reason for this peculiar quality of the right hemisphere is not known. It is possible that reticulocortical or corticoreticular fibers are more dense in the right hemisphere, although there is no currently available pathologic evidence that this is true. For a thorough discussion of the theories of the inattention syndrome, see Weinstein and Friedland.[25]

Contralateral inattention to double simultaneous stimulation is seen with parietal lesions of either hemisphere. The damage to parietal tissue apparently reduces reticulocortical interaction on the damaged side, thus allowing the intact hemisphere an advantage in the stimulus rivalry.[5,9] Such patients will characteristically report not feeling the stimulation on the side opposite the lesion even though both sides were stimulated with equal intensity.

Many functional mood alterations can affect attention. Anxiety causes distractibility and difficulty concentrating; depression produces disinterest and reduced arousal. All such mood changes hinder performance on attention tasks and generally decrease attention.

SUMMARY

Attention results from an interplay among brain stem, limbic, and cortical activity that allows the patient to focus on a specific task to the exclusion of irrelevant stimuli. Both functional and organic illness can disrupt attention and cause a failure of attention. Assessment of attention must be done early in the mental status examination because the valid testing of many subsequent functions relies on its integrity. Inattention and distractibility can significantly impair a patient's performance on the more demanding tasks of new learning, calculating, and verbal abstraction.

REFERENCES

1. Ballard, JC: Computerized assessment of sustained attention: A review of factors affecting vigilance performance. J Clin Exp Neuropsychol 18:843–863, 1996.
2. Bender, MB: Perceptual interactions. In Williams, D (ed): Modern Trends in Neurology, Vol 5. Appleton-Century-Crofts, New York, 1970, pp 1–28.
3. Bisiach, E and Vallar, G: Hemineglect in humans. In Boller, F and Grafman, J (eds): Handbook of Neuropsychology, Vol 1. Elsevier Science Publishers, Amsterdam, 1988, pp 195–222.
4. Critchley, M: The Parietal Lobes. Edward Arnold & Co., London, 1953.
5. Denny-Brown, D, Meyers, J, and Hornstein, S: The significance of perceptual rivalry resulting from parietal lesions. Brain 75:433, 1952.

6. Ferro, J and Kertesz, A: Posterior internal capsule infarction associated with neglect. Arch Neurol 41:422, 1984.
7. Gainotti, G: Emotional behavior and hemispheric side of lesion. Cortex 8:41, 1972.
8. Heilman, KM, Valenstein, E, and Watson, RT: The neglect syndrome. In Frederiks, JAM (ed): Handbook of Clinical Neurology, Vol 1(45), Clinical Neuropsychology. Elsevier Science Publishers, Amsterdam, 1985, pp 153–183.
9. Heilman, KM, Watson, RT, and Valenstein, E: Neglect and related disorders. In Heilman, KM and Valenstein, E (eds): Clinical Neuropsychology. Oxford University Press, New York, 1993, pp 279–336.
10. Invik, RJ, et al: Mayo's Older Americans Normative Studies: WAIS-R norms for ages 56–97. The Clinical Neuropsychologist 6:1, 1992.
11. Kahn, E and Cohen, L: Organic driveness: A brainstem syndrome and an experience. N Engl J Med 210:748, 1934.
12. Lezak, MD: Neuropsychological Assessment. Oxford University Press, New York, 1995, p 371.
13. Magoun, H: The Waking Brain. Charles C Thomas, Springfield, IL, 1963.
14. Mesulam, M-M: A cortical network for directed attention and unilateral neglect. Ann Neurol 10:309, 1981.
15. Morecraft, RJ, Gevla, C, and Mesulam, M-M: Architecture of connectivity within a cingulo-fronto-parietal neurocognitive network for directed attention. Arch Neurol 50:279–284, 1993.
16. Oxbury, J, Campbell, D, and Oxbury, S: Unilateral spatial neglect and impairment of spatial analysis and perception. Brain 97:551, 1974.
17. Simpson, N, Black, FW, and Strub, RL: Memory assessment using the Strub-Black Mental Status Examination and the Wechsler Memory Scale. J Clin Psychol 42:147, 1986.
18. Smith, A: The series sevens subtraction test. Arch Neurol 17:18, 1976.
19. Umilta, C: Orienting of attention. In Boller, F and Grafman, J (eds): Handbook of Neuropsychology, Vol 1. Elsevier Science Publishers, Amsterdam, 1988, pp 115–193.
20. Watson, RT, et al: Neglect after mesencephalic reticular formation lesions. Neurology 24:294, 1974.
21. Watson, RT, Valenstein, E, and Heilman, KM: Thalamic neglect. Arch Neurol 38:501, 1981.
22. Wechsler, D: Manual of the Wechsler Adult Intelligence Test, ed 3. The Psychological Corporation, New York, 1997, pp 181–194.
23. Wechsler, D: Manual for the Wechsler Memory Scale, ed 3. The Psychological Corporation, New York, 1997, pp 135–191.
24. Weinberg, WA and Harper, CR: Vigilance and its disorders. In Brumback, RA (ed): Behavioral Neurology. Neurol Clin 11:59–78, 1993.
25. Weinstein, EA and Friedland, RP (eds): Hemi-inattention and hemispheric specialization. Advances in Neurology, Vol 18. Raven Press, New York, 1977.

LANGUAGE

Language is the basic tool of human communication and the basic building block of most cognitive abilities. Its integrity therefore must be established early in the course of mental status testing. If deficits are found in the language system, the assessment of cognitive factors such as verbal memory, proverb interpretation, and oral calculations becomes difficult, if not impossible.

Language disturbances are commonly seen in patients with focal or diffuse brain disease; in fact, *demonstration of a specific language disturbance is pathognomonic of brain dysfunction.* Language disturbances have been well studied, and a number of distinct clinical neuroanatomic syndromes have been described. These are important to the clinician because of the relationship of specific language syndromes to neuroanatomic lesions. The ability to communicate using language is such a critical function that any disruption thereof results in a significant functional handicap.

To assess language function the examiner must first develop a systematic approach to the evaluation and then become acquainted with the various classic syndromes of language impairment. Cerebrovascular accidents (strokes), brain tumors, trauma, dementia, and other brain lesions or diseases may all cause language disturbances. Such disturbances are not always easily characterized by a cursory examination, and a familiarity with testing and the patterns of language disruption will make the aphasic, alexic, and agraphic syndromes more understandable.

TERMINOLOGY

Dysarthria is a specific disorder of articulation in which basic language (grammar, comprehension, and word choice) is intact. Patients with dysarthria produce distorted speech sounds that have a variable degree of intelligibility.

Dysprosody is an interruption of speech melody (e.g., tone, accent, tempo). Speech inflection and rhythm are disturbed, resulting in speech that is monotonal, halting, and sometimes mistaken for a foreign accent.[42]

Apraxia (buccofacial or oral) is the inability to perform skilled movements of the face and speech musculature in the presence of normal comprehension, muscle strength, and coordination. When asked to show how they would blow out a match, patients with apraxia may have difficulty approximating a pucker, inhale instead of exhale, exhale vigorously without puckering their lips, or say the word "blow." Any of these errors would be classified as apraxic. Oral apraxia that is evident only when the patient attempts to produce speech sounds is called **verbal apraxia**.

Aphasia is a true language disturbance in which the patient demonstrates an impaired production and/or comprehension of spoken language. The basic aphasic defect is in higher integrative language processing, although articulation and praxis errors may also be present. Aphasia usually refers to a loss of language after brain damage, but **"developmental aphasia"** is used when a child has a specific delay in language acquisition disproportionate to general cognitive development.

Alexia is the term used to describe a loss of reading ability in a previously literate person. Alexia does not refer solely to a total loss of reading ability, but to any level of acquired disturbance in reading. Alexia is not synonymous with dyslexia, which is a specific developmental learning disorder of children who have normal intelligence but who experience unusual difficulty in learning to read.

Agraphia is an acquired disturbance in writing. It refers specifically to errors of language and not to problems with the actual formation of letters or poor handwriting. Disorders of spelling are also included in this disorder.

EVALUATION

The language system should be evaluated in an orderly fashion. Specific attention must be paid to spontaneous speech, comprehension, repetition, and naming. Verbal language should be evaluated, and then reading and writing should be assessed. A short period of systematic testing can usually identify and roughly characterize an aphasic deficit. Because patients with aphasia are always agraphic and frequently alexic, the testing of reading and writing may be abbreviated in these cases. In those who are not aphasic, reading and writing should be fully evaluated because alexia or agraphia, or both, may be seen in isolation. Language testing can be very comprehensive; for further information, the interested examiner is referred to the test batteries listed in Appendix 1.

Handedness

Because of the close alliance between handedness and cerebral dominance for language, *the patient's handedness should be determined before beginning for-*

mal language testing. First, ask the patient whether he or she is right- or left-handed. As many natural left-handers have been taught to write with their right hand, observation of the hand used for writing may not be an accurate reflection of natural handedness. Next, ask the patient to demonstrate which hand is used to hold a knife, throw a ball, stir coffee, and flip a coin. Also, ask the patient about any tendency to use the opposite hand for any skilled movement. In addition, a family history of left-handedness or ambidexterity is important because handedness and cerebral dominance for language are significantly influenced by heredity. The spectrum of handedness ranges from strong right-handedness to left-handedness.[25] Strong or exclusive unilateral handedness is much stronger in right-handed than in non-right-handed persons. Also, patients with a strong family history of left-handedness tend to be ambidextrous and not strongly one-handed.[31] A statement of the patient's handedness as well as the family history of handedness should be recorded.

Spontaneous Speech

Eliciting Speech Production

The first step in language testing is *to listen carefully to the patient's spontaneous speech.* If the patient offers none, open-ended questions should be asked in order to elicit speech production. Listening to the patient's spontaneous speech even briefly may provide invaluable information that cannot be obtained during more formal aspects of the language examination. It is wise to ask the patient to discuss relatively uncomplicated issues, such as "Tell me why you are in the hospital" or "Tell me about your work." This type of general conversational question affords the patient a familiar topic and usually elicits his or her best efforts. In contrast, questions that require a mere "yes" or "no" answer will not provide sufficient speech output for meaningful evaluation. Pictures may be used to stimulate speech, but these can restrict the range of language output because of the limitations of the specific stimulus.

Observing Spontaneous Speech

Several clinical observations must be made and noted while listening to the patient's spontaneous speech:

- Is speech output present?
- Is the speech dysarthric or dysprosodic?
- Is there evidence of specific aphasic errors (e.g., errors of syntax, word-finding pauses, abnormal words, or paraphasias)?

The most obviously abnormal output is the total lack of any speech, in which patients may make some vocalizations but no meaningful linguistic utterances. This reduced output may be due to severe dysarthria, apraxia (buccofacial), or true aphasia. Of slightly less severity is a specific aphasic disorder that is characterized by stereotyped output in which the patient repeats the same utterance in response to each question. The utterance is usually a nonsense word like "bica, bica" or "a dis, a dis, a dis." Patients with very restricted output can, however, often surprise the naive examiner by producing well-articulated curse words or short phrases when under emotional stress.

Types of Aphasic Speech

Aphasic language production is characterized by errors of grammatic structure, difficulty in word finding, and the presence of word substitutions (paraphasias). One common type of aphasic speech pattern has been classified as **nonfluent**.[8,24] Nonfluent output is sparse and effortful, contains primarily nouns (substantive words), is agrammatic, and contains frequent word-finding pauses. For instance, the nonfluent patient describing winter weather might say "ah, ah, chold . . . snow . . . freezing . . . ah, ah . . . cold."

At the other end of the spectrum of fluency is a group of patients with aphasia who produce an easily flowing speech that is remarkably empty of content and contains many abnormal words (e.g., paraphasias). **Paraphasias** are words that are either substitutions for the correct word (e.g., "I drove home in my pen") or contain substituted syllables (e.g., "I drove home in my lar"). The complete word substitution ("pen" for "car") is a verbal or semantic paraphasia. The syllable substitution ("lar" for "car'") is a phonemic or literal paraphasia. The substitution of a non-English or nonsense word is the neologistic (new word) paraphasia ("I drove home in my strub").

Fluent aphasic speech is an easily recognizable speech pattern. The output is fluent and is characterized by normal or excessive rate of word production, often with a distinct press of speech. Content words (nouns and verbs) are lacking, and, in contradistinction to nonfluent output, small grammatic words such as articles, conjunctions, and interjections prevail. The nouns and verbs are often paraphasic. Because of the difficulty in producing nouns, word-finding pauses may interrupt the easy flow of speech. A patient with fluent aphasia who was describing a picture of a man after a shipwreck said the following: "It is a . . . I can see it . . . it is near a cold and he has a . . . actually what has happened is part of a . . . the rest of it there is a man right here and he is cold being out there." Occasionally, the language of the patient with aphasia contains so many paraphasic errors that the discourse is virtually unintelligible and impossible to follow. The term "jargonaphasia" is used for this heavily paraphasic but fluent speech.

The expressive language of many patients with aphasia cannot be classified strictly according to fluency. *The primary goal in the evaluation of a brain-damaged patient is to recognize that the language production is in fact aphasic.* With experience, the examiner can accurately recognize aphasic language and can classify the patient's language output, which often provides important information about the locus of the brain lesion. Patients with nonfluent aphasia are likely to have an anterior left hemisphere lesion, whereas those with fluent aphasia usually have posterior lesions.[8] This anterior-nonfluent, posterior-fluent dichotomy holds true in about 85% of cases, but sometimes the reverse is true (i.e., posterior lesion occurring with nonfluent aphasia, or an anterior lesion with fluent aphasia).[7] *The classification of an aphasia does not depend on the output characteristics alone; a complete evaluation of all language functions is always indicated.*

Verbal Fluency

Verbal fluency refers to the ability to produce spontaneous speech fluently without undue word-finding pauses or failures in word searching. Normal speech requires verbal fluency in the production of responses and the formulation of spontaneous conversational speech. This ability is often impaired after brain injury, especially that associated with anterior left hemisphere lesions. On formal testing, patients with aphasia almost invariably demonstrate some impairment in fluency. Additionally, individuals with early dementia or clinically silent left hemisphere lesions who exhibit relatively normal expressive speech and no other signs of word-finding difficulty may show subtle deficits on fluency tests. Verbal fluency is a reflection of word-finding efficiency, and fluency testing evaluates the patient's ability to scan memory traces rapidly in a specific semantic or phonemic category and to produce a series of responses in a given time frame.

An overall impression of fluency is gained by listening to the patient's spontaneous speech, but subtle defects in fluency can be elicited only through specific fluency tests. Verbal fluency is typically evaluated by tabulating the number of words the patient produces within a restricted category (e.g., animal types or words beginning with a specific letter) and within a specified time limit. Two easily administered evaluations are the **Animal-Naming Test**[30] and the **FAS Test** (a controlled oral word association test).[14] Tests using semantic categories such as animal names or grocery items are more sensitive indicators of early dementia than those using words beginning with a specific letter, such as the FAS Test.[6] We therefore usually use animal naming in clinical testing, especially when a deterioration in general cognitive functioning is suspected.

DIRECTIONS: For **animal naming**, instruct the patient to recall and name as many animals as possible. Any animal from the zoo, farm, jungle, water, or house is acceptable, but the examiner should not suggest these various locations, as subcategory shifting is one of the main cognitive challenges of this test. Time the patient's performance for 60 seconds, encouraging him or her to continue whenever necessary. The score is the number of correctly produced animal names during the 60 seconds. Record the correct responses as well as any paraphasic productions.

SCORING: The normal individual should produce from 18 to 22 animal names during a 60-second period, with the expected variation being ±5 to

7.[30,51] Age is a statistically significant factor in the expected performance on this task. Normal individuals age 69 and under will produce approximately 20 animal names, with a standard deviation of 4.5. This level of performance drops to 17 ($\pm$2.8) in the 70s and to 15.5 ($\pm$4.8) in the 80s. Scores of less than 13 in otherwise normal patients under age 70 should raise the question of impaired verbal fluency; scores less than 10 in patients under age 80 are suggestive of a word-finding problem; in an 85-year-old, however, a score of 10 may be the lower limit of normal.

DIRECTIONS: The **FAS Test** consists of three separate, timed word-naming trials, using the letters "F," "A," and "S," respectively. The patient is instructed to name as many words as possible (not including proper names) that begin with the stipulated letter during each 60-second trial. The patient's responses are recorded, including any paraphasias and repeated words that were produced in the three trials. Different forms of the same word (e.g., short, shorter) count as separate responses.

SCORING: Normal people name from 36 to 60 words, with performance depending in part on age, intelligence, and educational level.[14] An inability to name 12 or more words per letter is indicative of reduced verbal fluency. Performance on this test should be cautiously interpreted in patients with under 10 years of formal education or intelligence quotients (IQs) of less than 85.

Comprehension

Assessing the comprehension of spoken language is the next step in the language evaluation. *Comprehension must be tested in a structured fashion, without reliance on the patient's ability to answer verbally.* The most common error in assessing comprehension is to ask the patient to answer general or open-ended questions. Such questions require the patient to construct complex verbal answers that test the integrity of the entire language system and not verbal comprehension in isolation. Comprehension testing should require the minimum verbal response necessary for the patient to demonstrate that he or she has understood the examiner. For example, a question such as "What was the weather like in January?" does not assess language comprehension in isolation, whereas one such as "Is it snowing out today?" does.

We use two methods of testing comprehension: pointing commands and questions that can be answered with a "yes" or "no" response. Testing the patient's ability to point to single objects in the room, body parts, or articles collected from the examiner's pockets (e.g., coins, comb, pencil, keys) is an excellent way to quantify single-word comprehension. This task may be increased in complexity by requiring that the patient point to an increasing number of objects in sequence (e.g., "Point to the wall, the window, and your nose"). Increase the number of objects until the patient consistently fails. The patient of average intelligence without aphasia should succeed in pointing to four objects or more. Because the patient with aphasia who has comprehension difficulty may still be able to point to one or two items accurately, it is important to continue testing until consistent failure occurs. This test provides an evaluation of single-word comprehension, auditory retention, and sequence memory. For clarity, the level of performance should be described accurately on the test form.

Next, a series of simple and complex questions that require only "yes" or "no" answers should be asked. For example, "Is this a hotel?" "Is it raining today?" "Do you eat breakfast before dinner?" Question content may be simple or complex, as necessary. Before testing, be sure that the patient can reliably indicate "yes" and "no." Many patients confuse these two responses and cannot answer accurately or nod or shake the head appropriately. Also, it is important to ask at least seven questions because correct responses can occur by chance alone 50% of the time with "yes" and "no" questions. Correct answers should alternate between "yes" to "no" randomly because of the tendency for brain-damaged patients to perseverate. It is not uncommon for such patients to answer "yes" to 10 consecutive questions without knowing the correct answer to any of them.

Many clinicians test language comprehension by asking patients to carry out *motor commands* such as "Show me how to light a cigarette" or "Stick out your tongue." If the patient correctly carries out such commands, he or she has certainly understood them; however, many patients with aphasia have significant apraxia and fail to follow the command correctly because of a problem in high-level motor integration and not because of poor verbal comprehension.

Repetition

Repetition of spoken language is linguistically and, to some extent, anatomically a distinct function. In certain types of aphasia, repetition may be either spared or involved in relative isolation. Therefore, it is clinically relevant to test this function specifically. Repetition is a complex process that can be affected by impaired auditory processing, disturbed speech production, or disconnection between receptive and expressive language functions.

DIRECTIONS: Testing should present material in ascending order of difficulty, beginning with single monosyllabic words and proceeding to complex sentences. The following list of items provides a suitable range of difficulty. The patient should be asked to repeat the word or sentence verbatim after the examiner.

TEST ITEMS
1. Ball.
2. Help.

3. Airplane.

4. Hospital.

5. Mississippi River.

6. The little boy went home.

7. We all went over there together.

8. The old car wouldn't start on Tuesday morning.

9. The fat short boy dropped the china vase.

10. Each fight readied the boxer for the championship bout.

SCORING: The examiner must listen for paraphasias, grammatic errors, omissions, and additions. Normal people and brain-damaged patients without aphasia can accurately repeat sentences of 19 syllables.[46] Performance is related to intelligence and educational level, but errorless performance is expected on these specific items.

Naming and Word Finding

The ability to name objects is one of the earliest acquired and most basic language functions. Naming ability stays remarkably stable over the decades, with 80-year-olds performing at the same level as 25-year-olds.[45] Very old persons (over 80) and relatively uneducated persons over 70, however, tend to demonstrate mild naming problems.[49] Naming ability is almost invariably disturbed in all types of aphasia.[30] Impaired naming ability is called **anomia**.

Word-finding difficulty, which is closely related to anomia, is a reduced ability to retrieve the nouns and verbs used in spontaneous speech. Specific word-finding problems can be detected by listening to the spontaneous speech of the patient with aphasia. Asking the patient to describe a picture that contains objects and actions usually brings out any word-finding defect.

Anomia may also be objectively tested with a confrontation naming test. In this task, the examiner points to a variety of objects or pictures of objects and asks the patient to name them. The examiner should select from 10 to 20 items. Several categories of objects should be used (colors, body parts, room objects, articles of clothing, and parts of objects). Various categories are chosen because some patients with aphasia have a curious inability to name objects in a specific category while maintaining adequate ability to name objects in other categories. Because the disruption of naming has varying degrees of severity, it is important to use uncommon (low frequency of usage) items as well as common (high frequency of usage) items. For example, "nose," "arm," and "floor" are common, high-frequency words, whereas "watch stem and crystal," "shin," and "coat lapel" are uncommon, low-frequency words. Many patients with aphasia will be able to name common objects quickly and accurately, only to show great hesitancy, paraphasia, and circumlocution with uncommon objects. Some patients obviously recognize

TABLE 5-1. Objects for Confrontation Naming in Ascending Order of Difficulty by Category	
Colors	*Body Parts*
Red	Eye
Blue	Leg
Yellow	Teeth
Pink	Thumb
Purple	Knuckles
Clothing and Room Objects	*Parts of Objects*
Door	Watch stem (winder)
Watch	Coat lapel
Shoe	Watch crystal (lens)
Shirt	Sole of shoe
Ceiling	Buckle of belt

the object and are able to demonstrate and describe its use but cannot name it. For example, a patient shown a door key responded with "Oh, you know . . . the thing used to get in the . . . you turn it to get in."

The 20 items in Table 5–1, listed in ascending order of difficulty, are suggested for evaluating naming ability. Normal individuals will know all items except the parts of objects; on this set of five words the average score is 4.5 (± 0.8). The examiner should note that the names for parts of objects are low-frequency words and will be frequently misnamed or not named by most patients with aphasia and those with early dementia. With experience, each examiner will develop a personal repertoire of items tailored to his or her own office and patient population.

Reading

Reading ability is one of the few aspects of mental status testing that is directly related to educational experience. It is important, therefore, to determine the patient's educational background before testing reading. Demonstrating an alexia (reading deficit) in a patient, only to discover that he or she has had just 3 years of formal education, is merely documenting the patient's illiteracy.

Both reading comprehension and reading aloud ability should be tested. Both are usually defective in the same patient, but either can be disturbed in isolation. If the patient is not aphasic, screen for alexia by having the patient read a paragraph from a newspaper or magazine. To test reading in patients with aphasia, begin with having them read aloud first short single words, then phrases, sentences, and finally paragraphs. If they succeed at the lower levels, then have the patients read the names of objects in the room or on display and point to them. Finally, have patients read questions that can be answered "yes" or "no" or ask them questions about what was written. For example, if the patient read the sentence "The boy and girl walked in the snow," the examiner could ask, "Did the boy go alone?" or "Was it raining when the boy and girl went for a walk?"

The examiner should note any syllable or word substitutions (paralexic errors), omitted words, and defects in comprehension. Occasionally, patients have visual field defects or problems in ocular motility. In such cases, the examiner must help the patient stay on the written line and ensure that the patient completes one line before starting another. Using careful observation and examination, the examiner can readily separate the patients with true alexia from those having problems with the mechanics of reading.

Writing

Writing must be tested in the same way as that used to test reading. *If the patient shows evidence of aphasia, he or she undoubtedly also has an agraphia.* **Agraphia** is diagnosed when a patient demonstrates basic language errors, gross spelling errors, or use of paragraphias (word or syllable substitutions). To test writing, first have the patient write letters and numbers to dictation. Second, ask the patient to write the names of common objects or body parts. Third, if patients can successfully write single words, ask them to write a short sentence describing the weather, their job, or a picture from a magazine. Asking patients to write their name is not always particularly meaningful because name writing may be preserved even in the presence of gross agraphia. In the literate patient without aphasia, the examination can begin with this sentence-writing task. Patients with aphasia who cannot write spontaneously may show residual writing ability when asked to write to dictation.

Writing often shows a misalignment, in which the written line slants upward or downward. This misalignment is an error in the mechanics of writing but is not an agraphia per se.

Spelling

Spelling is a complex, little-studied, higher-language function that is strongly associated with educational experience. For practical purposes, spelling can be evaluated by asking the patient to spell dictated words. Gross errors in spelling can be detected in bedside testing; if it is important to establish an actual level of competence, standardized achievement tests should be used (Appendix 1).

CLINICAL IMPLICATIONS
Cerebral Dominance

Approximately 90% of the population is considered definitely right-handed. *Of this 90%, more than 99% are strongly left hemisphere–dominant for language.*[10]

Because of this strong language dominance in right-handed individuals, *left hemisphere lesions frequently cause aphasia*, whereas right hemisphere lesions rarely result in such deficits (i.e., a crossed aphasia).[52]

Left-handed individuals (non-right-handers) have a far different pattern of cerebral dominance for language. Approximately 70% are left hemisphere–dominant, 13% are right hemisphere–dominant, and the remainder are mixed.[28] In individuals with a strong family history of left-handedness (non-right-handedness, or sinistrality), this mixed dominance tends to be more prominent. Strongly left-handed individuals with no history of familial sinistrality tend to have the strongest left hemisphere dominance for language of all left-handed individuals. Accordingly, damage to either hemisphere in a left-handed patient usually results in aphasia. Aphasia in a left-handed patient with a lesion in either hemisphere is less severe than that resulting from a similar lesion in the left hemisphere of a right-handed patient. *Knowing the patient's cerebral dominance for language is important for localizing lesions and for deciding the risk that neurosurgical procedures pose to language.* In cases in which documentation of hemispheric dominance for language is critical (e.g., a left-handed patient with a right middle cerebral artery aneurysm), an intracarotid Amytal injection (Wada test) at the time of angiography can often establish dominance.[48]

Aphasia Syndromes

The impairment of language secondary to brain damage is not a unitary process; all components of language can show variable disruption. The extensive study of right-handed patients with aphasia has resulted in a generally accepted schema of cortical regionalization of language. Because some features overlap among patients who demonstrate mixed aphasia, some aphasiologists do not believe that this traditional neurologic classification system is suitable for neurolinguistic research.[16,50] However, this classification system follows the classic anatomic pattern, is easy for the student to understand, and is useful to the clinician for localizing lesions.

The clinical features of a patient's aphasia change dramatically over time. The acute destructive lesion causes maximal language disruption and is often associated with considerable disorientation and confusion. In the first several weeks, recovery is rapid and the aphasic picture constantly changes. After approximately 3 to 4 weeks, the aphasic pattern is more stable and may be fully assessed. The final prognosis of language recovery, however, cannot be given at that time because the reorganization and recovery process can continue for months or even years.

The posterior language area (area 1, Fig. 5–1) *is the cortical area primarily concerned with the comprehension of spoken language.* This area has traditionally been referred to as Wernicke's area, although the exact boundaries of the region have not been established.[12] *The anterior language area* (area 2, see Fig. 5–1) *subsumes the functions of language production.* Brodmann's area 44 within

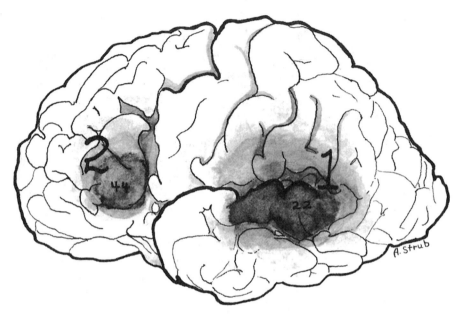

FIGURE 5-1. Anterior and posterior language areas.

the anterior language area is the classic Broca's area. Recent positron emission tomography (PET) studies of glucose metabolism have supported this regional specialization in patients with aphasia but have demonstrated that almost all such patients, irrespective of clinical characteristics, have evidence of hypometabolism in the temporal region on the left.[35] Such studies demonstrate that *the language system is quite complex physioanatomically* and is not simply a collection of cortical centers that act independently.

Traditionally, patients with damage in the posterior speech area are said to have "receptive aphasia" because of their primary difficulty in understanding spoken language. Patients with lesions in the anterior area are said to have "expressive aphasia" because of their primary difficulty in producing language. The problem with using "expressive aphasia" in this context, however, is that all patients with aphasia have *some* type of abnormal language expression. For this reason, we prefer to use the classification system described hereafter rather than the expressive-receptive dichotomy.

Global Aphasia

Global aphasia, the most common and severe form of aphasia, is characterized by spontaneous speech that is either absent or reduced to a few stereotyped words or sounds (e.g., "ba, ba, ba" or "dis, a dis, a dis"). Comprehension is absent or reduced to only recognition of the patient's name or a few selected words. Performance on repetition is at the same level as spontaneous speech. Reading and writing are likewise severely impaired. *Global aphasia is caused by a large lesion that damages most or all of the combined language areas 1 and 2* (anterior and posterior shaded areas). The most common lesion causing global aphasia is an occlusion of the internal carotid artery or the middle cerebral artery at its origin, caused by an embolus from the heart or carotid artery. Unfortunately, the prognosis for language recovery in these patients is poor. Global aphasia is almost always associated with hemiplegia. Because of these combined deficits, such patients have a severe chronic disability.

Broca's Aphasia

Patients with Broca's aphasia have nonfluent, dysarthric, dysprosodic, effortful speech. They utter mostly nouns and verbs (high-content words), with a paucity of grammatic fillers. The characteristic speech has been called agrammatic or telegraphic. For example, one patient with Broca's aphasia described a picture of a boy on a stool stealing cookies while his mother is washing dishes and letting the sink run over[30] in the following manner: "Boy . . .ah girl cookie . . . stool falling . . . water spilling . . . dishes." Repetition and reading aloud are as severely impaired in these patients as is their spontaneous speech. Auditory and reading comprehension are surprisingly intact, although the comprehension of complex grammatic phrases (e.g., "Do you eat lunch before breakfast?") is often impaired. Naming may show paraphasic responses.

This characteristic nonfluent aphasic syndrome results from a lesion in the anterior speech area (area 2, see Fig. 5–1). The lesion causing Broca's aphasia includes more than Brodmann's area 44 alone. Lesions restricted exclusively to area 44 result in only transient dysarthria or dysprosody.[3,36] Auditory and visual (reading) comprehension are intact because parietal and temporal lobes are not damaged. Patients with Broca's aphasia usually have right hemiplegia.

These patients often undergo an interesting and significant emotional change, characterized by frustration, agitation, and depression.[9] Whether this emotional change is a psychologic reaction to the loss of speech or a specific organic change associated with left frontal lobe damage is not yet known.[44]

The prognosis for language recovery in patients with Broca's aphasia is generally more favorable than in those with global aphasia. Because of relatively intact comprehension, these patients adjust better to life situations.

Wernicke's Aphasia

Wernicke's aphasia can be considered the linguistic opposite of Broca's aphasia. *The patient with Wernicke's aphasia has fluent, effortless, well-articulated speech. The output, however, contains many paraphasias and is often devoid of substantive words.* Patients often feel very pressed to speak. The following is an example of speech in Wernicke's aphasia. The patient was a ferry boat captain with a left temporal lobe brain tumor. In describing his previous work, the patient said, "Yea, I walked on the . . . always over . . . then pull it in . . . tie the . . . ah, ah over and back over wellendy catch it. . . ." The spontaneous speech can range from comprehensive sentences with occasional paraphasic errors to totally incomprehensible jargon in which most words are paraphasic and the output is devoid of content (jargonaphasia).

The essential feature of Wernicke's aphasia is a severe disturbance of auditory comprehension. Because the comprehension defect is so marked, the patient answers questions inappropriately and is completely unaware that the answers are often total nonsense. Repetition is severely impaired because of a severe auditory processing defect. Naming is grossly paraphasic. Reading and writing are also markedly impaired.

The lesion that causes Wernicke's aphasia is in the posterior language area (area 1, see Fig. 5–1). The more severe the defect in auditory comprehension, the more likely it is that the lesion involves the posterior portion of the superior temporal gyrus. If single-word comprehension is good but comprehension of complex material and written language is impaired, the lesion is more likely to involve the parietal lobe rather than the superior temporal lobe.[30] If the lesion also involves the middle and inferior temporal gyri, anomia is likely to be significant and persistent.[3] Because the damage is restricted to parietal and temporal lobes in most patients, the person with classic Wernicke's aphasia does not have hemiplegia.

Patients with Wernicke's aphasia are sometimes initially considered to be psychotic rather than aphasic. This confusion arises because the patient usually does not have a hemiplegia or other neurologic signs and produces inappropriate, but often reasonably well-formed, sentences. The gross comprehension deficit may not be appreciated, and the inappropriate answers to the examiner's questions are judged to be due to a basic thought disorder rather than a language disorder.

These patients often develop unusual patterns of behavior. They are frequently totally unaware of their problem and may talk endlessly without the slightest appreciation of their language deficit. This indifference may approach the point of euphoria. Other patients, however, develop a pronounced paranoid attitude accompanied by combative behavior.[9] This behavioral change may become chronic and require use of major psychotropic medication or treatment in a long-term psychiatric facility.

Patients with severe comprehension deficits do not have a good prognosis for language recovery, even with intensive language therapy. Milder Wernicke's aphasia may evolve into conduction or anomic aphasia, in both of which auditory comprehension is adequate but output contains paraphasias and word-finding pauses.

Conduction Aphasia

The hallmark of conduction aphasia is a disproportionate deficit in repetition. This syndrome is characterized by fluent, yet halting, speech with word-finding pauses and literal paraphasias. Comprehension is good, naming is mildly disturbed, and repetition is severely defective. This syndrome demonstrates that repetition and propositional speech (everyday language used to describe events or thoughts) are distinct psycholinguistic processes that can be selectively impaired by focal brain lesions. In conduction aphasia, reading is quite good, but writing shows errors in spelling, word choice, and syntax.

Two lesions are known to cause conduction aphasia. The first is usually reported to involve the supramarginal gyrus and arcuate fasciculus, a long fiber tract between the anterior and posterior areas (Fig. 5–2). The second

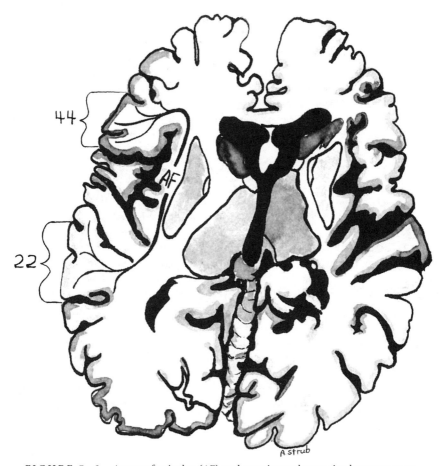

FIGURE 5–2. Arcuate fasciculus (AF) and anterior and posterior language areas.

lesion damages the insula, contiguous auditory cortex, and underlying white matter. This lesion spares the arcuate fasciculus, which arches higher into the parietal operculum.[21] This entity represents one of the clinical disconnection syndromes[23] because it literally disconnects the auditory sensory cortex from the motor speech cortex.

Transcortical Aphasias

The linguistic opposite of conduction aphasia is transcortical aphasia. *The transcortical aphasias are characterized by intact repetition of spoken language but disruption of other language functions.* Some patients have difficulty producing speech while having adequate language comprehension; others produce fluent speech but have poor comprehension.

The patient with transcortical motor aphasia can repeat, comprehend, and read well but has the same kind of restricted spontaneous speech exhibited by patients with Broca's aphasia. In contrast, the patient with transcortical sensory aphasia repeats well but does not comprehend what he or she hears or repeats. Spontaneous speech and naming are fluent but paraphasic, as in Wernicke's aphasia. Occasionally, a patient may have a combination of transcortical motor and sensory aphasias. These individuals can repeat long sentences, even in a foreign language, with remarkable accuracy. Repetition is very easy to initiate in these patients, even inadvertently, because some patients have a tendency to be echolalic (to repeat everything said within the range of their hearing).

The lesions that cause transcortical aphasia are either extensive, crescent-shaped infarcts within the border zones between major cerebral vessels (e.g., within the frontal lobe between the territories of the anterior and middle cerebral arteries and posteriorly between middle and posterior cerebral arteries [Fig. 5–3]) or subcortical lesions of the white matter underlying these areas of cortex. Transcortical motor aphasia is seen with an anterior border zone lesion, whereas transcortical sensory aphasia indicates a lesion that resembles a reversed C (see Fig. 5–3). These lesions spare the superior temporal and inferior frontal cortex (areas 22 and 44 and their immediate environs) and the parietal perisylvian cortex. This spared perisylvian cortex is all that is required for complete and accurate language repetition. When this region is the only language area spared by combined border zone infarcts, the resulting language deficit (echolalia) has been called the "isolation of speech syndrome."[26] The most common causes of the transcortical aphasias are (1) anoxia secondary to decreased cerebral circulation, as seen in cardiac arrest; (2) occlusion or significant stenosis of the carotid artery; (3) anoxia due to carbon monoxide poisoning; and (4) dementia.[13,43]

Recovery from transcortical sensory aphasia is relatively good, but few data are available regarding the prognosis in the motor or mixed transcortical aphasias.

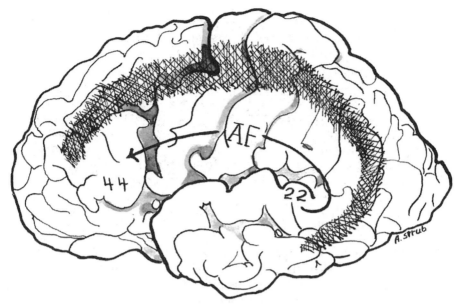

FIGURE 5-3. Border zone infarct that produces transcortical aphasia.

Anomic Aphasia

In some patients with aphasia, the only language defects are word-finding difficulty and an inability to name objects on confrontation. This condition has been labeled anomic, nominal, or amnestic aphasia. Spontaneous speech is usually fluent and grammatically rich but contains many word-finding pauses and paraphasias of specific object names. Auditory comprehension is very good, except when the patient is asked to point to a series of specific objects. This comprehension defect is a result of two-way dissociation of naming: the patient cannot name objects and frequently has difficulty recognizing object names when offered in examination. Repetition is good, with the exception of sentences that contain many nouns. Reading and writing may be impaired in specific patients; the degree of alexia and agraphia depends entirely on the location of the lesion that is responsible for the aphasia.

Lesions in many parts of the dominant hemisphere can cause anomic aphasia; thus, the localizing significance of this type of aphasia is limited. Neurosurgical mapping studies of naming have demonstrated multiple sites where naming can be interrupted with a low-level electric current.[40] The sites differed widely among patients, and the only area that produced naming problems in more than 50% of the patients was the posteroinferior frontal cortex. The most severe anomic aphasia, however, is noted in patients with temporal lobe lesions involving the second and third temporal gyri. This area cannot be considered an actual "word dictionary" but includes important pathways from the occipital lobe to the limbic system that are critical for object naming.[23] Lesions in the parietotemporal area also result in rather severe anomia. Patients with these lesions also have significant alexia with agraphia. Accordingly, the combined syndrome of alexia and agraphia with anomic aphasia localizes a lesion to the left parietotemporal area.

Anomias may be so mild that they are scarcely detectable in normal conversation or so severe that spontaneous output is nonfluent and devoid of meaningful content. The prognosis for language recovery depends on the severity of the initial defect. Because language output is relatively spared and comprehension reasonably intact, such patients make better life adjustments than other, more severely affected, patients with aphasia.

Subcortical Aphasia

Some patients with vascular lesions (either hemorrhage or infarct) of the thalamus, putamen caudate, or internal capsule will demonstrate aphasic symptoms. These individuals are dysarthric and often run words together in their speech. They have mild anomia and comprehension deficits but excellent repetition.[20,37] Anterior lesions tend to produce speech-production problems, whereas posterior lesions result in comprehension difficulty.[38]

The mechanisms by which these subcortical lesions produce aphasia are not clear.[17] In some cases, the disorder seems more a motor-speech problem; in others, a true aphasia or language disturbance is present.[32] Because the cortex is thought to be the repository of language engrams, it is most likely that the subcortical damage alters the input to and function of the overlying cortex. In one study of glucose uptake in patients with aphasia caused by subcortical lesions, Metter and associates[34] demonstrated a definite decrease in cortical metabolism in addition to the expected decreased metabolism of the subcortical structures.

Aphasia in Left-Handed Individuals
(Non-Right-Handers)

Owing to their mixed cerebral dominance, *left-handed individuals may become aphasic secondary to a lesion in either hemisphere.* The resultant aphasia is usually milder and is associated with greater recovery than an aphasia caused by a similar lesion in a right-handed patient. In 35% to 40% of these cases, the aphasia cannot be classified within the traditional scheme. Wernicke's aphasia or the agrammatism of Broca's aphasia is rarely seen. Decreased verbal fluency and dysarthria are common, but comprehension and repetition are usually relatively intact. Naming and reading are defective when the lesion is in the left hemisphere.[15,27]

Crossed Aphasia

Crossed aphasia refers to the rare cases in which a right-handed individual develops an aphasia from a *right* hemispheric lesion. In 70% of such cases, the patients demonstrate a language syndrome similar to that of left hemisphere–dominant right-handers;[5] in the other 30% of cases, however, syndromes and signs vary widely.[4]

Language in Alzheimer's Disease

A progressive deterioration in language facility is observed in atrophic (cortical) dementia. In the earliest stage, the patient's conversation wanders in a circumlocutory fashion and can be difficult to follow. The content of conversational speech is simplified and reflects the general decrease in intellectual ability. Word-finding pauses may be present and verbal fluency is reduced. As the disease progresses, word-finding difficulty becomes prominent and paraphasic substitutions are seen. Spontaneous speech lacks relevance and may be tangential. Intrusions of words or phrases from earlier parts of a conversation may appear at inappropriate times. Comprehension is also decreased. Naming is reduced and may be paraphasic. Repetition, however, is preserved quite late in the course of the dementia.

In the late stages of the disease, there is little spontaneous speech or comprehension. Echolalia is often seen. In the final decorticate state, the patients become mute.[1,18]

Progressive Aphasia

An interesting progressive language disorder called **progressive aphasia** is caused by relatively restricted left frontotemporal degeneration. Such patients usually show a slowly progressing nonfluent aphasia and apraxia, with good preservation of comprehension and other cognitive functions for many years. Many of them eventually become demented in the late stages of their illness. Pathologically, these cases are mixed: some show findings of Alzheimer's disease; some, Pick's disease; and some, Creutzfeldt-Jakob spongiform encephalopathy or other degenerative disorders.[11,33]

Pure Word Deafness

Pure word deafness is a rare syndrome in which patients do not have aphasic speech, agraphia, or alexia, yet are lacking in verbal language comprehension. In these patients, hearing is intact and nonlanguage sounds (auditory gnosis) are recognized.

The lesion that produces this condition is located in the posterior language area and is often bilateral. The lesion is deep in the temporal lobe and effectively disconnects auditory input from the auditory cortex.[2]

Articulation Disturbances

Dysarthria

Pure dysarthrias are caused by a disruption in any of the inputs to the muscles of articulation: the cortex, as in Broca's aphasia; the basal ganglia, as in parkinsonism or cerebral palsy; bilateral striatal or pontine lesions, as in pseudobulbar palsy; or the bulbar neurons, as in amyotrophic lateral sclerosis. The patient with pure dysarthria can communicate normally using reading and writing.

Buccofacial Apraxia

Buccofacial apraxia may be caused by various lesions between the supramarginal gyrus and the frontal lobe in the dominant hemisphere. Lesions in these areas appear to interrupt the motor planning necessary for the complex movements of normal speech. Many patients with aphasia, particularly Broca's or conduction aphasia, have considerable apraxia of facial movement. Some patients with language output resembling Broca's aphasia may, in fact, have pure buccofacial apraxia. The difficulty in separating the aphasic and apraxic components of speech in some patients has lead some speech pathologists to consider Broca's aphasia as merely a motor-speech disorder and not a true aphasia. Broca's aphasia can be seen, however, in the absence of any buccofacial apraxia. Therefore, *careful examination of each patient is important to separate the apraxic and aphasic components.*

Dysfluency

Dysfluency (stuttering or stammering) is another speech-production problem. Not an aphasia, apraxia, or dysarthria, it is a common speech disorder whose exact etiology is not known, although mixed dominance is seen in many cases. Both organic and functional explanations have been advanced. *Dysfluency is usually a developmental speech disorder, but it can be acquired secondary to a brain lesion.*

Alexia

Several distinct syndromes exist in which reading ability is impaired secondary to acquired brain lesions. *The classic syndrome of pure alexia without agraphia*[22,23] *is caused by a left posterior cerebral artery occlusion in a right-handed individual.* The resulting cerebral infarct damages the posterior portion of the corpus callosum as well as the left occipital lobe. Because the left visual cortex is damaged, all visual information enters only the right hemisphere. The right visual cortex perceives the written material but cannot transmit it to the left hemisphere because of the callosal lesion (Fig. 5–4). The inferior parietal lobule in the dominant hemisphere (primarily area 39, the angular gyrus) is the association cortex that combines the visual and auditory information necessary for reading and writing. In alexia without agraphia, the inferior parietal lobule is disconnected from all visual input. Because the lobule and its connections within the language area are intact, the patient can write normally. One of the dramatic aspects of this syndrome is the patients' ability to write lengthy, meaningful messages, only to be unable to read his or her own writing. These patients are able, however, to understand words spelled aloud. Interestingly, most patients with this syndrome can name objects and discuss

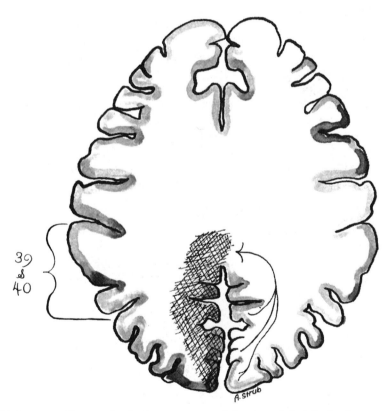

FIGURE 5–4. The cross-hatched area represents infarction of the left visual cortex and the posterior portion of the corpus callosum. The visual information from the right visual cortex *(arrow)* is unable to reach the left inferior parietal lobule (39 and 40) because of the callosal lesion.

visual events that are occurring in their environment. This type of visual information must cross to the left hemisphere by some pathway other than the damaged posterior corpus callosum.

A second distinct type of alexia, classically called alexia with agraphia, *results from damage to the inferior parietal lobule itself (angular gyrus and environs). This lesion renders the patient unable to read or write.* These patients are not appreciably aphasic but may have a certain degree of anomia. Recognition of this syndrome is clinically important for localization; in the right-handed patient with this syndrome, the lesion is invariably in the left inferior parietal area. The most common acquired alexia is neither of the pure syndromes but rather the alexia associated with aphasia.

Agraphia

Writing is a complex motor task that involves the translation of a language item into written symbols.[29] The linguistic message to be written originates in the posterior language area, is then translated into visual symbols in the inferior parietal area, and is finally transferred to the frontal language area for motor processing. Lesions within any of these language areas will cause an agraphia. With the exception of patients with pure word deafness, *all patients with aphasia show some degree of agraphia.* Although the most common agraphia is the form that is accompanied by aphasia, under certain circumstances agraphia may be seen in the absence of aphasia.

Two syndromes are seen in patients with damage to the dominant parietal lobe: (1) agraphia with alexia, described in the previous section; and (2) a syndrome of agraphia in association with other parietal lobe signs (dyscalculia, right-left disorientation, and finger agnosia), called Gerstmann's syndrome (discussed in detail in Chapter 9).

One rare pure agraphia occurs only in the left hand. This syndrome is seen in patients with lesions of the anterior corpus callosum. These patients are agraphic with the left hand only, because the right motor cortex is disconnected from the language areas of the left hemisphere. Writing with the right hand is normal because of the intact connections of the left motor cortex and the language areas. Figure 5–5 demonstrates the normal pathways required for writing. The callosal lesion (F_1) appears to interrupt the language message going to the right hemisphere.

Single case reports describe isolated pure agraphia resulting from superior parietal lesions.[47]

Psychotic Language (Bizarre Language Output)

Rambling, disjointed, neologistic language can be seen in patients with severe psychosis (especially schizophrenia), advanced organic dementia, delirium, and fluent

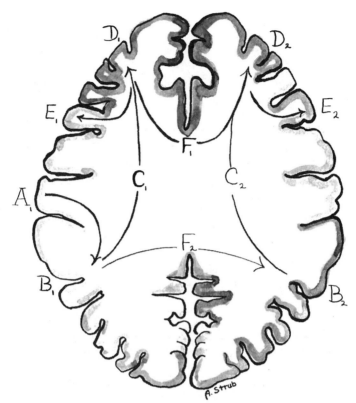

FIGURE 5-5. The written message originates in the posterior language area of the dominant hemisphere (B_1). The message is transferred via the arcuate fasciculus (C_1) to the premotor area in the same hemisphere (D_1). Motor patterns are transferred to the motor strip (E_1) for innervation of the right hand. The message must cross via the anterior corpus callosum (F_1) to the right motor system (D_2, E_2) for innervation of the left hand. F_2 is not a significant pathway for transferring the written message to the right motor area.

jargonaphasia. Differentiation among these conditions on the basis of spontaneous speech alone may be difficult. Historical data are invaluable: in elderly persons an acute onset of gross language disturbance with aphasia or delirium favors the diagnosis of a stroke; a prolonged history of language deterioration in the young patient indicates schizophrenia or an unusual organic lesion such as a left hemisphere glioma; a gradual deterioration of language in the older patient suggests dementia or a focal brain lesion such as a left hemisphere tumor or subdural hematoma. Unfortunately, detailed historical information is often unavailable, and a tentative diagnosis must at such times be based on mental status findings alone.

Each of the aforementioned conditions has certain features that help to distinguish it from the others. Systematized paranoid delusions may be seen in both aphasia and dementia, but are much more common in schizophrenia. Neologisms are used infrequently by patients with schizophrenia, but their use is usually consistent and symbolic (e.g., one patient with paranoid schizophrenia repeatedly referred to the "frinky-franks" that were placed in the walls to watch him). Neologisms produced by patients with aphasia tend to be random, very frequent, and nonsymbolic (e.g., "The walret is the you know, wimbit, lep, olla other one"). Those with dementia often have word-finding difficulty and produce circumlocutory speech with some paraphasias. Until the late stage of the dementia, their speech is generally more comprehensible and less paraphasic than that of the patient with aphasia. The patient with advanced dementia produces little speech, and what is produced may be largely neologistic isolated words or short neologistic word strings.

Because it is difficult to differentiate among these conditions by listening to spontaneous speech alone, complete language testing is essential. Careful comprehension testing reveals that patients with jargonaphasia are unable to understand even very simple commands. Delirious, moderately demented, or schizophrenic patients have adequate comprehension but may be difficult to evaluate because of a lack of cooperation. Patients with aphasia usually demonstrate inferior performance in repetition testing. Naming tasks clearly reveal language problems in patients with aphasia by their production of paraphasic errors. A patient with aphasia who is shown a key may say, "Pel, klo, klep, kleep . . . key," whereas one with schizophrenia may call it a "key sort of watching tower thing." In this instance, the patient with schizophrenia correctly identified the object but incorporated it into his or her disordered thought process. Patients with delirium or dementia usually have some naming trouble but not as severe as that seen in patients with aphasia nor as bizarre as that seen in those with schizophrenia. When asked to name a key, the patient with dementia might well answer, "Lock, no . . . the lock keyer . . . key!"

The differential diagnosis of these conditions is important because a misdiagnosis may lead to gross mismanagement. For example, we saw a very robust 80-year-old retired grocer who began answering questions inappropriately at dinner one evening. Becoming concerned, his wife continued to ask questions, which the husband was unable to answer. He became frustrated, angry, and agitated. The wife became frightened and called the police. Because of this aggressive behavior, the man was jailed for 3 days. He was then transferred to a psychiatric hospital, where he remained for an additional 3 days before a neurologist diagnosed a Wernicke's aphasia secondary to a middle cerebral artery thrombosis. Mistakes such as this can be made unless a careful mental status examination is performed.

Differentiating patients with dementia from those with schizophrenia is usually not difficult because of the age at onset, differences in behavior, and distinct differences in verbal output. On complete examination, additional data may corroborate the initial opinion. The patient with dementia may show problems with praxis and drawing. The patient with schizophrenia often distorts drawings but usually can make recognizable copies of designs and figures. Ideational apraxia (Chapter 9), which can be demonstrated by asking the patient to fold a letter and place it in an envelope, is often present in patients with dementia but not in those with schizophrenia.

Nonorganic Speech and Language Disorders

Several types of functional speech disorders can be mistaken for organic language patterns. Some neurotic patients convert anxiety into a halting, effortful, telegraphic speech pattern (e.g., "Me want go home see wife"). These patients have normal comprehension, repetition, and naming but reduced verbal fluency. Reading and writing are also intact but are carried out in the same slow, effortful fashion. Mild dysarthria may also be present. These patients may require the help of psychiatrists and speech pathologists to alter their speech patterns.

Other functional patients develop an acute aphonia (total inability to adduct the vocal cords and make audible sounds). Aphonia may arise as a pure conversion symptom or, more commonly, secondary to an insult to the speech apparatus. One middle-aged patient remained aphonic for 2 months after awakening from surgery with an endotracheal tube in place. Aphonic patients breathe normally and show no evidence of stridor (a sign of vocal cord paralysis). They communicate well by gesture, mouthing words, and writing. This type of functional overlay is well known to speech pathologists and responds well to therapy.

Elective mutism is another functional speech disorder that may be seen in both children and emotionally disturbed adults. It is characterized by a willful reluctance or an outright refusal to speak. The disorder may be complete (i.e., an absolute lack of speech in all situations) or relative (i.e., selective communication with a small circle of intimates). The speech, when present, may be limited to a mouthing of words; whispering; or a slow, labored, halting production. The adult who elects to remain mute typically has no language deficit and is physiologically capable of producing speech sounds. Some patients, especially children, do have a basic organic language disorder with considerable emotional overlay. The mutism is often resistant to the usual forms of speech therapy and psychotherapy[41] but can respond to behavior modification.[39]

SUMMARY

Language is a very complex and interesting higher-cognitive function. Because of the unique relationship of language and cerebral dominance, most acquired language disorders are pathognomonic of left hemisphere damage.

Careful evaluation of language functions can localize the lesion within the dominant hemisphere. Language is critically important for many other cognitive functions; thus, the subsequent parts of the mental status examination must be administered and interpreted with some caution in patients with aphasia.

REFERENCES

1. Albert, ML: Language in normal and dementing elderly. In Obler, LV and Albert, ML (eds): Language and Communication in the Elderly. Lexington Books, Lexington, MA, 1980, pp 145–150.
2. Albert, ML, et al: Clinical Aspects of Dysphasia. Springer-Verlag, Vienna, 1981, pp 88–91.
3. Alexander, M: Aphasia: Clinical and anatomic aspects. In Feinberg, TE and Forah, MJ (eds): Behavioral Neurology and Neuropsychology. McGraw-Hill, New York, 1997, pp 133–149.
4. Alexander, MP and Annett, M: Crossed aphasia and related anomalies of cerebral organization: Case reports and a genetic hypothesis. Brain Lang 55:213–239,1996.
5. Alexander, MP, Fischett, MR, and Fischer, RS: Crossed aphasia can be mirror image or anomalous. Brain 112:953–973, 1989.
6. Barr, A and Brandt, J: Word-list generation deficits in dementia. J Clin Exp Neuropsychol 18:810–822, 1996.
7. Basso, A, et al: Anatomoclinical correlations of the aphasias as defined through computerized tomography: Exceptions. Brain Lang 26:201, 1985.
8. Benson, DF: Fluency in aphasia: Correlation with radioactive scan localization. Cortex 3:373, 1967.
9. Benson, DF: Psychiatric aspects of aphasia. Br J Psychiatry 123:555, 1973.
10. Benson, DF and Geschwind, N: Cerebral dominance and its disturbances. Pediatr Clin North Am 15:759, 1968.
11. Benson, DF and Zaias, BW: Progressive aphasia: A case with postmortem correlation. Neuropsychol Behav Neurol 4:215, 1991.
12. Bogan, J: Wernicke's area: Where is it? Thoughts about (and against) cortical localization. Paper presented at the 13th Annual Meeting of the Academy of Aphasia. Victoria, BC, October 5, 1975.
13. Bogousslavsky, J, Regli, F, and Assal, G: Acute transcortical mixed aphasia: A carotid occlusion syndrome with pial and watershed infarcts. Brain 111:631, 1988.
14. Borkowski, JG, Benton, AL, and Spreen, O: Word fluency and brain damage. Neuropsychologia 5:135, 1967.
15. Brown, JW and Hécaen, H: Lateralization and language representation. Neurology 26:183, 1976.
16. Caramazza, A: The logic of neuropsychological research and the problem of patient classification in aphasia. Brain Lang 21:9, 1984.
17. Crosson, B: Subcortical Functions in Language and Memory. The Guilford Press, New York, 1992.
18. Cummings, JL and Benson, DF: Dementia: A Clinical Approach. Butterworth & Co, Boston, 1983.
19. Damasio, AR: Aphasia. N Engl J Med 326:531, 1992.
20. Damasio, AR, et al: Aphasia with nonhemorrhagic lesions in the basal ganglia and internal capsule. Arch Neurol 39:15, 1982.
21. Damasio, H and Damasio, AR: The anatomical basis of conduction aphasia. Brain 103:337, 1980.
22. Dejerine, J: Des differentes varietes de cecite verbale. Mémoires de la Société de Biologie 1892, pp 1–30.
23. Geschwind, N: Disconnection syndromes in animals and man. II. Brain 88:585, 1965.
24. Geschwind, N: Current concepts in aphasia. N Engl J Med 284:654, 1971.
25. Geschwind, N and Galaburda, AM: Cerebral Dominance: The Biological Foundations. Harvard University Press, Cambridge, MA, 1984.

26. Geschwind, N, Quadfasel, F, and Segarra, J: Isolation of the speech area. Neuropsychologia 6:327, 1968.
27. Gloning, K: Handedness and aphasia. Neuropsychologia 15:355, 1977.
28. Goodglass, H: Understanding Aphasia. Academic Press, San Diego, 1993.
29. Goodglass, H: Disorders of writing. In Goodglass, H: Understanding Aphasia. Academic Press, San Diego, 1993, pp 172–192.
30. Goodglass, H and Kaplan, E: The Assessment of Aphasia and Related Disorders, ed 2. Lea & Febiger, Philadelphia, 1983.
31. Hécaen, H and de Ajuriaguerra, J: Left Handedness: Manual Superiority and Cerebral Dominance. Grune & Stratton, New York, 1964.
32. Luria, AR: On quasi-aphasia speech disturbances in lesions of the deep structures of the brain. Brain Lang 4:432, 1977.
33. Mendez, MF and Zander, BA: Dementia presenting with aphasia: Clinical characteristics. J Neurol Neurosurg Psychiatry 54:542, 1991.
34. Metter, EJ, et al: Comparison of metabolic rates, language and memory in subcortical aphasias. Brain Lang 19:33, 1983.
35. Metter, EJ, et al: Cerebral glucose metabolism in Wernicke's, Broca's and conduction aphasia. Arch Neurol 46:27, 1989.
36. Mohr, JP: Broca's area and Broca's aphasia. In Whitaker, H and Whitaker, H (eds): Studies in Neurolinguistics, Vol 1, Perspectives in Neurolinguistics and Psycholinguistics. Academic Press, New York, 1976, pp 201–235.
37. Mohr, JP, Watters, WC, and Duncan, AW: Thalamic hemorrhage and aphasia. Brain Lang 2:3, 1975.
38. Naeser, MA, et al: Aphasia with predominantly subcortical lesion sites: Description of three capsular/putaminal aphasia syndromes. Arch Neurol 39:2, 1982.
39. Norman, A and Broman, H: Volume feedback and generalization techniques in shaping speech of an electively mute boy: A case study. Percept Mot Skills 31:463, 1970.
40. Ojemann, G, et al: Cortical language localization in left dominant hemisphere: An electrical stimulation mapping investigation in 117 patients. J Neurosurg 71:316, 1989.
41. Reed, G: Elective mutism in children: A re-appraisal. J Child Psychol Psychiatry 4:99, 1963.
42. Ross, ED: Nonverbal aspects of language. In Brumback, CA (ed): Behavioral Neurology. Neurol Clin 11:9–23, 1993.
43. Rubens, AB and Kertesz, A: The localization of lesions in transcortical aphasias. In Kertesz, A (ed): Localization in Neuropsychology. Academic Press, New York, 1983, pp 245–268.
44. Strub, RL: Mental disorders in brain disease. In Frederiks, JAM (ed): Handbook of Clinical Neurology, Vol 2(46), Neurobehavioral Disorders. Elsevier, Amsterdam, 1985, pp 413–441.
45. Tombaugh, TN and Hubley, AM: The 60-item Boston Naming Test: Norms for cognitively intact adults aged 25 to 80 years. J Clin Exp Neuropsychol 19:922–932, 1997.
46. Vargo, ME and Black, FW: Normative data for the Spreen-Benton Sentence Repetition Test. Cortex 20:585, 1984.
47. Vignolo, LA: Modality specific disorders of written language. In Kertesz, A (ed): Localization in Neuropsychology. Academic Press, New York, 1983, pp 357–369.
48. Wada, J: A new method for the determination of the side of cerebral speech dominance: A preliminary report on the intracarotid injection of sodium amytal in man. Med Biol 14:221, 1949.
49. Welch, LW, et al: Educational and gender normative data for the Boston Naming Test in a group of older adults. Brain Lang 53:260–266, 1996.
50. Willmes, K and Poeck, K: To what extent can aphasic syndromes be localized? Brain 116:1527–1540, 1993.
51. Wilson, RS, Kaszniak, AW, and Fox, JH: Remote memory in senile dementia. Cortex 17:41, 1981.
52. Zangwill, OL: Two cases of crossed aphasia in dextrals. Neuropsychologia 17:167, 1979.

CHAPTER

6

MEMORY

A disturbance in memory is the most common cognitive complaint of patients with organically based behavioral syndromes. *Almost all patients with dementia show memory problems early in the course of their disease.* In dementia the problem is insidious and can make it difficult or impossible for patients to function effectively. They may lose track of the date, forget work details, or fail to remember commitments extending beyond their daily routines. This can have devastating effects on patients' social and vocational life, especially before the nature of the problem is fully appreciated. Recognition of this memory difficulty allows the clinician and the family to help these patients to avoid potential personal catastrophe. *Careful attention to memory testing often reveals the presence of an organic disorder before abnormal findings are noted on standard neurologic examination.*

Various neurologic diseases result in different types of memory disturbance (e.g., severe memory deficit in relative isolation in Korsakoff's syndrome, memory difficulty compounded by inattention and agitation in the confusional states, impaired recent memory associated with general cognitive dysfunction in dementia). In each of these diseases, memory is disturbed by different pathophysiologic mechanisms.

Not all memory difficulties have neurologic origins. Depressed and anxious patients, as well as other patients with significant psychiatric disorders, often have difficulty with memory. Because performance on memory testing requires maximum patient cooperation and effort, the emotionally disturbed patient often performs poorly. The misdiagnosis of depression as dementia or the reverse is a serious diagnostic error that can lead to months or even years of inappropriate treatment. Untangling the memory problems in patients with a psychiatric disorder is difficult; however, full neurologic, psychiatric, and psychologic evaluation can almost always lead to the correct diagnosis. The diagnostic challenge is even greater when a problem such as early Alzheimer's disease is compounded by a superimposed depression or anxiety.

TERMINOLOGY

Memory is a general term for a mental process that allows the individual to store information for later recall.[33] The time span for recall can be as short as a few seconds, as in a digit repetition task, or as long as many years, as in the recall of one's childhood experiences.

The memory process consists of three stages. In the first stage, the information is *received and registered* by a particular sensory modality (e.g., touch, auditory, or visual). Once the sensory input has been received and registered, that information is held temporarily in short-term memory (working memory). The second stage consists of *storing or retaining* the information in a more permanent form (long-term memory). This storage process is enhanced by repetition or by association with other information that is already in storage.[25] Storage is usually an active process requiring effort through practice and rehearsal.[23] Some information, however, is stored passively throughout our lives; this process is called **incidental memory** because it is acquired effortlessly. The final stage in the memory process is the *recall, or retrieval,* of the stored information. This retrieval is an active process of mobilizing stored information on request or as needed (so-called declarative memory).

Each stage in the total memory process relies on the integrity of the previous stages. Any interruption in the hierarchy may prevent the storage or retrieval of a memory. Formal studies of memory have demonstrated that each aspect of memory involves separate yet interlocking neurobiologic substrates or systems. The effects on these systems differ according to the patient's particular disease, and each produces a different clinical picture.

Clinically, memory is subdivided into three types, based on the time span between stimulus presentation and memory retrieval. "Immediate," "recent," and "remote" are commonly used to denote these basic memory types. Unfortunately, these terms are nonspecific, and the time span each implies is not well defined in clinical use. Immediate memory, or **immediate recall**, is used to recall a memory trace after an interval of a few seconds, as in the repetition of a series of digits. Sometimes **short-term memory** is also used to describe this memory type, when the recall interval is filled with a distractor such as having the patient count backward.

Recent memory is the patient's capacity to remember current, day-to-day events (e.g., the current date, the doctor's name, what was eaten for breakfast, or recent news events). More strictly defined, recent memory is the ability to learn new material and to retrieve that material after an interval of minutes, hours, or days.

Remote memory traditionally refers to the recall of facts or events that occurred years previously, such as the names of teachers and old school friends, birth dates, and historic facts. In patients with a specific defect in new learning (recent memory), remote memory refers to the recall of events that occurred before the onset of the recent memory defect.

Amnesia is a general term for a defect in memory function. Although applied to a broad spectrum of memory defects, amnesia is used most commonly to label patients with severe and relatively isolated memory deficits (e.g., Korsakoff's syndrome or posttraumatic amnesia). The inability to learn new material *after* a brain insult is called **anterograde amnesia**. The inability to remember events that occurred *before* the brain insult is called **retrograde amnesia**. The period of amnesia in either case may be as short as a few seconds or as long as several years. It is most commonly seen with head trauma but may also follow any major brain insult (e.g., stroke). Amnesia may also refer to **psychogenic amnesia**, in which the patient blocks a period of time from memory. These patients do not demonstrate a recent memory deficit, can learn items during the amnestic period, and, after the amnestic period is over, do not have a defect in recent memory when tested. Psychologically based memory loss leaves patients with gaps, or relative gaps, in their memory for the events that occurred during the amnestic period. Sometimes patients recall parts of the amnestic period that were not emotionally traumatic while blocking recall of the traumatic events themselves.

EVALUATION

In the mental status examination, each aspect of memory should be assessed in some detail. This allows the examiner to distinguish the type of memory deficit (if any), the degree of memory loss, and the impact of the memory deficit on the patient's ability to function.

Patients commonly perform at different levels on various memory tests, depending on the nature of the disorder (e.g., patients with Korsakoff's syndrome can respond very adequately to questions regarding remote events but cannot learn new material). The use of several different memory tests is also of clinical importance. Brain-damaged patients demonstrate differences in the incidence, nature, and degree of memory deficits based on the type of test used and the nature and location of their lesions.[2,3,9,17]

The accurate assessment of memory requires that any question asked by the examiner be verifiable from a source other than the patient. For example, it is useless to ask patients when they graduated from high school or what they ate for lunch if the examiner cannot ascertain the accuracy of the patients' responses. Many patients with readily demonstrable memory deficits deny their problem and may confabulate answers. Such responses may appear perfectly appropriate to the naive examiner who is unable to verify their accuracy. Personal information concerning the patient's social history, lifestyle, vocation, and so forth should be verified by the patient's family or friends.

Historic facts (e.g., "When was World War II?" or "Who was the President before Mr. Clinton?") are commonly used by examiners to screen both remote and recent memory. Because the knowledge of such information is closely related to the patient's basic premorbid intellectual level, education, and general social exposure, the examiner must be mindful of these factors when considering the use of historic facts to test memory. If used at all, questions related to historic material must be tailored to the patient's background.

The most sensitive and valid tests of recent memory are those that require the patient to learn new material and recall it over time. The use of this technique eliminates some of the dangers of encountering unverifiable material and unknown social background. New learning is an active memory process that requires more expenditure of effort by the patient than does the mere recall of personal or historic facts.

When evaluating memory, the examiner must be aware of various factors that can impair performance even in individuals who do not have an organic memory deficit. Because memory test performance requires the patient's sustained attention, inattentive, distractible patients cannot perform optimally on such tests, regardless of the etiology of their memory problem. Patients in an acute confusional state or who have a severe psychogenic disorder usually have impaired attention, which hinders memory test performance. Disturbances of basic sensory, motor, or language functions that interfere with comprehension or expression also cause impaired memory test performance. Poor memory performance by patients who are deaf, aphasic, acutely confused, psychotic, anxious, depressed, or grossly inattentive may reflect defects caused by these processes alone and should not be interpreted as evidence of an underlying memory deficit. *Valid memory testing presumes that the patient is reasonably attentive, can relate to and cooperate with the examiner, and has no defect that impairs language comprehension or expression.* Any evidence of aphasia, whether a subtle residual effect of a more significant aphasia (e.g., after a stroke) or a mild defect noted on examination, impairs both short-term and long-term verbal memory.[38] Extreme caution must be exercised when interpreting a verbal memory impairment in such patients.

Because of the clinical and social importance of memory, we have selected a number of memory tests that enable the examiner to assess a variety of memory processes. Many patients become apprehensive when having their memory tested, so it is important to present the material slowly and in as calm and nonthreatening a fashion as possible.

Immediate Recall (Short-Term Memory)

Immediate recall is usually tested by digit repetition, which was covered in detail in Chapter 4 and will not be repeated here. Although backward digit repetition has been used by some examiners to assess verbal memory, this is a highly complex task that requires several neuropsychologic processes in addition to memory.[4] It is useful as a general screening test for brain dysfunction but should not be considered a test of short-term memory in isolation.

Orientation (Recent Memory)

The patient's orientation with respect to person (who he or she is), time (the date), and place (where he or she is) is important preliminary information and should be evaluated early in the examination of memory functioning.

Orientation to place and time are actually measures of recent memory, as they test the patient's ability to learn these continually changing facts. If a patient is not fully oriented, this alone suggests a significant recent memory deficit.

DIRECTIONS: The patient should be asked the following questions in sequence. Questions may be paraphrased when necessary to ensure clarity. If the patient fails these items, tell the patient the correct answers and have him or her repeat them; several minutes later, have the patient recall the answers. Failure at this level verifies poor new learning ability and predicts deficient performance on any subsequent memory tasks.

TEST ITEMS

1. Person	
a. Name	What is your name?
b. Age	How old are you?
c. Birth date	When is your birthday? (day, month, year)
2. Place	Where are we right now?
a. Location	What is the name of this place?
	What kind of place are we in now?
	What floor did you come to today?
b. City location	What city are we in now?
	State? County?
c. Address	What is your home address?
3. Time	
a. Date	What is today's date? (year, month, date)
b. Day of the week	What day of the week is it?
c. Time of day	What time is it right now?
d. Season of the year	What season is it now?

SCORING: Normal people usually perform perfectly on this test, with some individuals receiving somewhat less adequate scores on time orientation.[29] The only items sometimes failed by normal individuals are the exact date of the month and, less commonly, the day of the week. Performance correlates with education level; normal college graduates, if they do not know the exact date or day, usually miss by only 1 day, whereas normal people without a high school education may miss by 2 or even 3 days.[22] A small number (7.7%) of normal uneducated individuals may incorrectly identify the month.

Remote Memory

Remote memory tests such as those included here evaluate the patient's ability to recall personal and historic events. As previously emphasized, personal events must be verifiable by a reliable source other than the patient, and performance on the recall of historic information must be interpreted in light of the patient's premorbid intelligence, education, and social experience.

TEST ITEMS

1. Personal information
   a. Where were you born?
   b. School information | Where did you go to school?
   When did you attend school?
   Where is your school located?
   c. Vocation history | What do you do for work?
   Where have you worked?
   When did you work at those places?
   d. Family information | What is your wife's (children's) name?
   How old is your wife (children)?
   What was your mother's maiden name?

SCORING: Personal information items are completed with approximately equal accuracy by both normal patients and patients with mild, nonspecific brain damage. Although impaired performance is pathologic, this test does not efficiently differentiate among groups.[29]

TEST ITEMS AND SCORING

Historic facts:

Ask the patient to name four people who have been president during the patient's lifetime. The normal patient should be able to accomplish this task without difficulty. A slightly more difficult task, and one that is very frequently failed by patients with early Alzheimer's disease, is asking the patient to name the last four or five presidents in proper reverse sequence, starting with the current president.

Ask the patient to name the last war in which the United States was directly involved. At the time of this writing, the correct response would be the war in Iraq (Desert Storm). An older patient may name the Vietnam War, Korean War, or World War II. If the patient gives one of these responses, ask him or her about any recollection of the Iraq war. If the patient has no memory for these major events, this implies deficient memory.

New-Learning Ability

This section assesses the patient's ability to actively learn new material (to acquire new memories). Adequate performance requires the integrity of the total memory system: recognition and registration of the initial sensory input, retention and storage of the information, and recall or retrieval of the stored information. An interruption in any of these stages impairs clinically relevant new-learning ability. A careful clinical examination of how a patient fails a particular task may often provide valuable information as to the nature of the impaired process. Patients with impaired memory, particularly those with Alzheimer's disease, can become rather overwhelmed during extensive memory testing. Items previously presented inhibit and confuse learning on subsequent items (proactive interference). In such situations, the patients may provide answers from earlier test items in later testing. These intrusion errors are characteristic of many organic syndromes, especially dementia.

Four Unrelated Words

DIRECTIONS: Tell the patient, "I am going to tell you four words that I would like you to remember. In a few minutes, I will ask you to recall these words." To ensure that the patient has heard, understood, and initially retained the four words, have him or her repeat the words after their presentation. Correct any errors made on immediate repetition. Older patients (over age 75) may require several trials to learn the words, but when a patient must be given four or five trials to repeat the words accurately, this usually forecasts a significant memory problem. To eliminate possible mental rehearsal, interference should be used between presentation and recall of the words. Accordingly, the examiner may wish to present the four words before the remote memory or orientation examination. After 5 minutes, ask the patient to recall the four words. Information concerning the duration of memory can be obtained by asking for another recall of the words after 10 and 30 minutes. The following sets of words have been selected because of their semantic and phonemic diversity. Only one set of words should be used with a given patient, because of possible contamination and resultant confusion.

TEST ITEMS

1. Brown	1. Fun	1. Grape
2. Honesty	2. Carrot	2. Stocking
3. Tulip	3. Ankle	3. Happiness
4. Eyedropper	4. Loyalty	4. Toothbrush

When a patient cannot recall a given word, it is often possible to obtain an indication of memory storage by the use of verbal cues. These include semantic cues relating to the category of the named object (e.g., "One word was a color"), phonemic cues using syllabic components of the word (e.g., "Hon . . . [honesty]"), and contextual cues (e.g., "A flower"). If a patient cannot recall the words either spontaneously or with cues, the examiner may resort to asking the patient if he or she recognizes the appropriate word from a series of words (e.g., "Was the color red, green, brown, or yellow?"). When this yields significantly better results than spontaneous recall, the memory problem may be due to a retrieval defect rather than to an acquisition or storage deficit. This demonstration of good memory on recognition testing but poor memory on free recall is called **implicit memory**.

SCORING: The normal patient under age 60 should accurately recall three or four of the words after a 10-minute delay.[29] Normal results for this test

	Normal Individuals (Age in Years)					Alzheimer's Disease Patients (Stage)			
	40–49	*50–59*	*60–69*	*70–79*	*80–89*	*I*	*II*	*III*	*IV*
4 Words									
5 min	3.1	2.9	2.0	1.8	2.1	1.6	0.4	0	0
	(0.9)	(1.3)	(1.0)	(0.8)	(1.4)	(1.2)	(0.7)	(0.1)	
10 min	3.7	3.5	3.0	2.6	2.7	1.9	0.7	0.1	0
	(0.7)	(0.8)	(1.0)	(0.9)	(1.4)	(1.4)	(1.0)	(0.4)	
30 min	3.7	4.0	3.5	3.1	2.9	1.8	0.6	0.1	0
	(0.7)	(0.0)	(0.7)	(1.2)	(1.1)	(1.4)	(1.0)	(0.3)	
Story	10.1	11.1	9.7	8.2	7.6	5.5	2.8	0.6	0
	(2.8)	(1.9)	(2.6)	(3.3)	(2.8)	(2.3)	(2.0)	(1.0)	
5 Objects	4.6	4.7	4.2	3.9	3.8	2.3	1.1	0.2	0
	(0.6)	(0.6)	(0.8)	(1.0)	(1.6)	(1.7)	(1.3)	(0.5)	
Paired Associate Learning (Both Trials)									
Easy	3.8	3.8	3.6	3.1	3.6	3.2	2.4	0.8	0
	(0.4)	(0.6)	(0.7)	(1.2)	(0.7)	(0.7)	(0.9)	(1.1)	
Difficult	3.3	3.2	2.6	2.1	2.3	1.7	0.9	0.1	0
	(1.0)	(0.7)	(1.3)	(1.0)	(1.0)	(0.9)	(1.0)	(0.4)	

TABLE 6–1. **Recent Memory Performance***

*Mean and standard deviation, n = 100.

vary significantly (standard deviation 0.8 words), however, so the clinical implication of a low score (e.g., 2 of 4) must be interpreted in light of the patient's history and the performance on the entire examination. As shown in Table 6–1, an age-related decline in performance on this test is seen in normal individuals over age 60. Normal persons over age 80 retain an average of only two of four words over 5 minutes, with a substantial variance. After being reminded of the correct words, these individuals will improve their performance after 10 and 30 minutes. Patients with dementia, on the other hand, tend not to improve on subsequent trials.

Verbal Story for Immediate Recall

DIRECTIONS: Tell the patient, "I am going to read you a short paragraph. Listen carefully, because when I finish reading, I want you to tell me everything that I told you." For older patients, read the story more slowly to give them adequate time to process the information. After reading the story, say "Now tell me everything that you can remember of the story. Start at the beginning of the story and tell me all that happened." The separate items in the story are indicated by slash (/) marks. As the patient retells the story, indicate the number of items recalled. In patients with good immediate recall, it may be useful to ask for another recall after 30 minutes. This is a sensitive method of assessing short-term verbal recall.

TEST ITEM

It was July / and the Rogers / had packed up / their four children / in the station wagon / and were off / on vacation.

They were taking / their yearly trip / to the beach / at Gulf Shores. / This year / they were making / a special / one-day stop / at the Aquarium / in New Orleans.

After a long day's drive / they arrived / at the motel / only to discover / that in their excitement / they had left / the twins / and their suitcases / in the front yard.

SCORING: The story contains 26 relatively separate ideas or information bits. In our experience, the normal individual under age 70 should be expected to produce at least 10 of these items on immediate recall. For patients in their 70s, the average score drops to 8.2, and in their 80s, to 7.6. Elderly individuals are slower in their auditory processing and less able to store as much information on a single presentation as are younger people. Less adequate performance than that shown by age-specific values (see Table 6–1) by the nonretarded patient indicates defective verbal recall ability. Story recall significantly discriminates between normal individuals and Alzheimer patients and also between brain-damaged and low-IQ normal groups (Tables 6–1 and 6–2, respectively).

TABLE 6-2. **Statistical Comparison of Memory Tests**

Variable	Brain Damaged Mean	Low-IQ Normal Mean	F
Total score	33.4	50.0	28.0‡
Digit repetition	4.2	4.8	1.9
Vigilance errors	10.2	0.2	5.5†
Orientation	8.7	10.6	13.3‡
Person	2.6	3.0	7.5‡
Place	2.7	3.0	3.4*
Time	3.4	4.6	8.4‡
Remote memory			
Personal information	3.4	3.9	3.1
Historic facts	1.3	1.5	3.2
Four words—10 min	1.9	3.6	15.1‡
Four words—30 min	1.8	3.9	20.4‡
Visual memory			
Hidden objects found (4)	1.3	3.7	10.8‡
Hidden objects named	1.0	0.2	3.1
Paired associate learning			
Easy	2.1	3.0	12.6‡
Difficult	1.4	3.0	9.7‡
Total	3.5	6.0	15.6‡

*$P < .05$.
†$P < .01$.
‡$P < .001$.

Visual Memory (Hidden Objects)

Visual memory should be tested in all patients, but it is especially useful in evaluating the memory of patients with aphasia. It is also a good nonthreat-ening test to use for patients whose history has already indicated considerable memory problems or for those with reduced verbal abilities or lack of education.

DIRECTIONS: The examiner may use any five small, easily recognizable objects that may be readily hidden in the patient's vicinity. We commonly use items such as a pen, comb, keys, coin, and fork. The use of five items provides a reasonable span for most patients. The objects are hidden while the patient is watching. Name each item as it is hidden to ensure that the patient is aware of which object was hidden in what place. After hiding the objects, the examiner should provide interfering stimuli for 5 minutes by administering another mental status task, asking the patient routine ques-tions, or engaging the patient in general conversation. After this period, ask the patient to name and indicate the location of each of the hidden objects. If the patient cannot recall the location of any object, ask him or her to name the hidden object.

SCORING: The average patient under age 60 should find four or five (4.6 ± 0.6) of the hidden objects after a 5-minute delay without difficulty. Older patients (age 70 to 90) will not do quite as well (3.8 ± 1.3). Less adequate performance (fewer than three objects) indicates impaired visual memory. A patient with aphasia should be able to find and demonstrate the use of the objects but may not be able to name them.

Paired Associate Learning

Paired associate learning (PAL) is commonly used in standard memory bat-teries and is another highly sensitive measure of new-learning ability.

DIRECTIONS: Tell the patient, "I am going to read you a list of words, two at a time. Listen carefully because I will expect you to remember the words that go together. For example, if the words were 'big' and 'little,' I would expect you to say the word 'little' after I said the word 'big.' " When the patient understands the directions, continue as follows: "Now listen carefully to the words as I read them." Read the first presentation at the rate of one pair every 2 seconds. After reading the first presentation, test for recall by presenting the first recall list. Give the first word of a pair and allow 5 seconds for a response. If the patient gives a correct response, say "That's right" and proceed with the next pair. If the patient gives an incorrect response, say "No," provide the correct word, and proceed to the next pair.

After the first recall has been completed, allow a 10-second interval and give the second presentation list, proceeding as before.

TEST ITEMS

PRESENTATION LISTS

First Presentation	*Second Presentation*
Weather—Box	House—Income
High—Low	Weather—Box
House—Income	Book—Page
Book—Page	High—Low

RECALL LISTS

First Recall	*Second Recall*
House—	Book—
High—	House—
Weather—	High—
Book—	Weather—

SCORING: The normal patient under age 70 is expected to recall the two "easy" paired associates (high—low, book—page) and at least one of the "hard" associates of the first recall trial, and to recall all paired associates on the second trial. In patients over age 70, performance is slightly less adequate.[26] Some patients can learn the paired words with strong natural associations but cannot learn the pairs without such associations. This discrepancy demonstrates a reliance on semantic cues and an inability to learn new material that cannot be associated with memories already in storage. The total PAL score is the best measure of verbal learning.

The results of a statistical comparison of these memory tests between 25 patients with mixed brain damage and 25 normal patients with IQs less than 80 appear in Table 6–2. Differences in age and education were controlled.[29]

CLINICAL IMPLICATIONS

Some aspects of the memory process are associated with certain neuroanatomic structures or neuronal systems. Pathologic studies have amply documented that limbic structures are involved in the long-term storage and retrieval of recent information.[7,21,26,36] However, the structures required for immediate recall and remote memory are not as well established. Although all memory traces—visual, verbal, tactile, and polymodal—are most likely stored in the neocortex, many subcortical structures are necessary for the total memory process (registration, storage, and retrieval). *Damage or disruption of different cortical or subcortical systems result in varied patterns of dysfunction.*

Immediate Recall

The immediate recall of digits is a process that does not require any long-term storage of information but does require initial registration, short-term holding, and verbal repetition. This entire process can be performed by the language cortex surrounding the sylvian fissure, as demonstrated in patients with transcortical aphasia.[13] The exact mechanism by which these short-term memories are maintained within the language system is not known. Reverberating circuits may be established, or patterns of cortical after-image may be present. Whatever change does occur, however, is not long-lasting.

Efficient short-term memory is not a passive process, and several factors favor good performance. A digit-sequence task is performed much better if active mental rehearsal can take place. Also, if the patient actively groups digits into two- or three-digit sets, performance will be improved. A third and always very important element in all memory processing is the association of the new material with previously stored information; for example, a digit sequence that is similar to an old phone number or address will be much more easily recalled than a completely unique random sequence. Short-term memory (immediate recall) is a distinct property of the cortical sensory, motor, and integrative areas necessary to register, recall, and produce the original stimulus. *It does not require the limbic system, as do long-term storage and permanent memory formation.*

If these basic sensory or motor areas are damaged or disrupted, then short-term memory will be faulty. In digit repetition, the language system is essential, so any degree of aphasia (excluding the transcortical aphasias) can disrupt immediate memory functioning. This repetition failure is particularly pronounced in conduction aphasia,[35] the primary deficit of which is an inability to repeat. Whether this repetition failure is a defect of language or short-term memory is an open question that may, in fact, reflect an argument of semantics.

The most common cause of failure on short-term memory tasks is probably inattention.[30] If a patient's attention strays from the stimulus during presentation, the information may be imperfectly registered. Similarly, if the patient is inattentive during the repetition phase and pauses occur, the memory trace will fade. Inattention can be organic, as in confusional states and dementia, or functional, as in anxiety and depression.

Patients with dementia have difficulty with immediate memory for several reasons: such patients are often inattentive; they have cortical atrophy, which affects their basic language and other sensory-motor integration systems; and they have general intellectual deterioration.[39]

Recent Memory

In general, the ability to store and then retrieve new material (recent memory, new learning, or memorizing) presumes intact registration, retention, and short-term storage. If the material is familiar and can be associated with information already in long-term storage, the process is easier and relies less on short-term storage.[25]

Certain limbic structures are required to ensure storage and retrieval. The medial temporal lobe, the mamillary bodies, and the dorsal medial nuclei of the thalami are essential subcortical links in the storage and retrieval of both verbal and nonverbal memories.[7,26,36] The degree of memory loss is related to the extent of damage within this system. When there is bilateral temporal lobe damage, injury to the hippocampus is sufficient to produce memory problems; if there is also damage to the subiculum and the perihippocampal and entorhinal cortices, the memory loss becomes profound.[40] Actual memories are probably not stored in these structures, but the limbic system seems to act as the mechanism to store and retrieve memories from the cortex. Frontal lobe damage (primarily affecting the orbital cortex) also can impair recent memory; this situation is most commonly seen after rupture of an anterior communicating artery aneurysm.

Whenever these subcortical structures are destroyed or severely damaged, the patient is rendered unable to learn new material (anterograde amnesia) or to retrieve memories from the recent past (retrograde amnesia). These patients literally become fixed in time and are unable to record the passing of events from that time onward. *If these limbic structures are damaged in isolation (i.e., with no additional damage outside the limbic system), patients develop a profound organic amnesic state.* This condition is characterized clinically by (1) severe anterograde amnesia; (2) moderate to severe retrograde amnesia, which can extend back for several years; and, usually, (3) confabulation during the acute stage. In the face of this devastating memory impairment, such patients have remarkably intact immediate memory, as assessed by digit repetition and similar tests. These patients also demonstrate no change in premorbid levels of intelligence. They carry on coherent, intelligent conversations that appear abnormal only when recent events are discussed. Because these patients do not remember the date, place, and recent events, they may appear confused.

This dramatic amnesic state has been seen secondary to bilateral temporal lobectomy, herpes simplex encephalitis, and bilateral hippocampal infarction in which the hippocampi have been completely destroyed. A similar memory deficit is seen clinically in Korsakoff's syndrome (a syndrome of thiamine depletion seen in chronic alcoholism and severe malnutrition), in which there is bilateral destruction of the mamillary bodies and the dorsal medial nuclei of the thalami. The patient with Korsakoff's syndrome frequently, but not invariably, goes through an acute encephalopathy (Wernicke's encephalopathy) at the onset of the memory difficulty. Vascular or traumatic lesions of the dorsal medial thalamus also cause severe organic amnesia.[16,31,34] The patient with Korsakoff's syndrome shows good implicit memory; that is, the patient can recognize if he or she has seen a previously presented item, rather than recalling or retrieving it from memory. This implicit memory is strictly a cortical process, in which the memory trace has been stored without the patient's awareness.[10,27]

In Alzheimer's dementia, patients also have defects in new learning, which are due in part to a gradual degeneration of the cells in the hippocampus and in the basal nucleus of Meynert. The memory loss in the atrophic dementias is more complex than that seen in the organic amnesias, and it is discussed more fully in the section on remote memory.

The amnesia most familiar to the lay person is the memory loss that occurs after head injury. *Patients with moderate to severe closed head injury almost always have some degree of retrograde amnesia for the time immediately preceding the injury, and they usually have transient difficulty learning new material after the trauma (anterograde amnesia).* In head trauma, the temporal lobes are commonly concussed against the bony confines of the middle fossa. This trauma causes a physiologic disruption of hippocampal function, which in turn disturbs memory storage and retrieval. Posttraumatic amnesia is usually reversible, but in cases of significant temporal lobe damage, the memory loss can be permanent. Repeated concussion, such as that seen in boxers, may result in gradual but permanent memory disturbance. An interesting feature of the amnesia seen with acute head injury is that the retrograde amnestic period will shorten in the days following recovery of consciousness. Initially the patient may not recall events that occurred years preceding the accident. Within several days, the patient may remember all but the few minutes that immediately preceded the accident. This shrinking retrograde amnesia verifies that the injury did not eliminate the memories from storage but merely rendered them temporarily irretrievable.[1,18] In some interesting trauma cases retrograde amnesia is profound and persistent even after the anterograde amnesia clears.[19] Such cases indicate that neuroanatomic subsystems exist for the various aspects of recent memory.

Clinically, the memory disturbance in the various types of organic amnesias is similar (i.e., the patients cannot recall recent information). On experimental tasks, however, it has been shown that patients with Korsakoff's syndrome, whose damage is in the thalamus and mamillary body, have actually retained a considerable amount of the material presented to them, but are unaware of this (the memory is implicit but not explicit). The deficit is with retrieving the information and realizing that it has been presented, rather than with the storage process. Patients with hippocampal and temporal lobe damage have both a storage and a retrieval defect. As mentioned earlier, the fact that the cortex of the patient with Korsakoff's syndrome has stored the engrams for the memory does not help the patient clinically because he or she does not realize that they are stored and thus cannot retrieve and use the information.[37]

Transient global amnesia is another type of organic memory problem.[15] *This syndrome probably involves transient ischemia of both medial temporal lobes secondary to decreased perfusion in the territory of the posterior cerebral arteries.*[14,20] Single photon emission computerized tomography (SPECT) perfusion scans usually demonstrate this bilateral or unilateral left temporal lobe hypoperfusion. This syndrome is characterized by an acute but temporary confusional state with amnesia. The patients are disoriented to time and place and have a significant defect in new-learning ability. Fortunately, recovery generally occurs within hours or days, and the patient is left with a permanent amnesia only for the duration of the episode itself. Some patients, however, may experience permanent memory loss and demonstrate bilateral hippocampal infarction.[8] The following case illustrates some of the essential features of this syndrome:

> Dr. JL was a robust 68-year-old educator who was addressing a teacher's convention. In the middle of his speech, he stopped suddenly, became dazed, and began to ask where he was. He repeatedly asked, "What am I doing?" and "Where am I?" On initial neurologic examination, he was distraught and very confused. He was unable to attend well, and he could not learn new material. He did not remember arriving in New Orleans, but he *did* know that he was scheduled to attend the convention. One day later, his mental function was essentially normal, except that he was amnesic for the day prior to and the day of his amnesic episode.

All of the conditions discussed thus far have resulted from bilateral lesions localized in limbic structures. *Although it is true that a bilateral lesion is necessary to produce a profound memory loss, there is some loss of specific memory functions after a unilateral lesion.* Patients who have had a unilateral dominant temporal lobectomy show a relative decrease in verbal learning, whereas those with unilateral nondominant temporal lobectomies show a decrease in visual memory.[21] This pattern of differential deficits is also seen with unilateral subcortical lesions.[32]

Various factors other than specific limbic damage can interfere with the storage and retrieval of new material; some of these have been discussed in the previous section, but they merit additional mention here. Inattention will prevent any patient from accurately storing new material. Because efficient memory storage requires close attention to the information for short-term registration and storage, the results of memory testing in inattentive patients must be interpreted with caution. Patients with aphasia are also at a tremendous disadvantage in any verbal learning task; if they cannot accurately comprehend or repeat verbal material, it is not valid to judge their memory capacity using that material. Nonverbal memory tasks are necessary for valid assessment of memory in patients with aphasia. Memory-test performance and intelligence are directly related; accordingly, patients' premorbid intellectual levels must be considered when interpreting the results of memory testing. Deficits in basic sensory capacity (i.e., hearing and vision) are sometimes overlooked in testing, but obviously sensory systems must be adequate for memory testing in each specific modality.

Certain medications are also well known to produce genuine memory deficits. Psychotropic drugs, beta blockers (e.g., propranolol), anticonvulsants, prednisone, and any number of other medications and toxins (e.g., alcohol and street drugs) have been implicated.

The patient's emotional state can also significantly affect new-learning ability. Very anxious patients often make errors owing to inattention and distractibility. Depressed patients perform poorly on memory testing because of their inability to put forth the required effort to memorize the presented material.

Depressed patients also tend to remember negative or sad events or ideas more effectively than they do positive or happy ones.[5] In significant depression, the decrease in motivation and learning probably involves more than purely psychologic mechanisms. The underlying chemical disorder postulated in major depressive disorders undoubtedly adversely affects neuronal functioning at various levels.[11]

Poor performance on memory tests is probably the single most important factor that may result in the misdiagnosis of depression as dementia.[24] Accordingly, in the patient with psychomotor retardation and memory problems, the diagnosis of depression must be considered and carefully pursued during the evaluation process.

Remote Memory

When a memory has remained in a person's repertoire for a number of years, it can be considered a remote, or old, memory. *Old memories are stored in the appropriate association cortex (e.g., language cortex for verbal material).* In contrast to recent memory, *remote memory does not require the limbic system for retrieval from storage.* Patients with Korsakoff's syndrome or bilateral temporal lobectomy can accurately discuss personal and historic events that occurred years previously (remote memory), yet they are unable to remember what they had for breakfast that morning (recent memory).[28] There is apparently a mechanism, thus far unexplained, by which memories finally become sufficiently well established that they can be recalled without the aid of subcortical limbic structures. These remote memories can be lost only by damage to the cortical storage areas themselves. *This loss of remote, or old, memories is seen in patients with the atrophic dementias (Alzheimer's and Pick's) or any disease that damages extensive areas of the cortex.* The memory disturbance in the patient with dementia is complex: such patients have difficulty with short-term memory because of atrophy in the basic sensory association cortex (e.g., language cortex for verbal memory); they are hampered in recent memory acquisition because of degeneration of cells in the basilar nucleus of Meynert and hippocampal system; and they have defects in remote memory because of widespread cortical atrophy.

Functional Memory Disturbances

Not all memory disorders are of organic origin, and knowledge of the functional disturbances of memory is important. The interference with memory performance that can occur secondary to anxiety and depression has been discussed previously. In addition, studies of Vietnam War veterans have demonstrated stable memory deficits in servicemen suffering from posttraumatic stress disorder.[5] *There are, however, several psychiatric conditions in which memory disturbances are central features. The first and most common is the dissociative state, now called psychogenic amnesia.* This is the classic amnesia that has been popularized in the press and in movies. Such patients either lose their identity completely and travel to a new location (fugue, psychogenic fugue state, or dissociative amnesia) or have periods of minutes, hours, or days when they carry out their normal life routine and later become aware that they remember nothing of what transpired during this period (dissociative state or localized amnesia). During a dissociative or fugue state, the patients do not usually act confused, as do persons with transient global amnesia, and they are able to learn new material, unlike patients with organic amnesia. *There should be no difficulty in differentiating patients with organic amnesia, who cannot learn new material when tested, from those with psychogenic amnesia, who have experienced a "memory lapse."* Brief testing using the Four Unrelated Words task or the PAL task should suffice.

One other curious pseudomemory disturbance is Ganser's syndrome, or the syndrome of approximate answers. These patients routinely give approximate answers to all questions: for example, saying that today is Tuesday (actually it is Wednesday), the month is March (actually it is April), or 2 and 2 are 5. Because their answers are so consistently close to the correct answer, it is obvious that they have more knowledge of the subject in question than they are indicating. Although giving the approximate answer is the most characteristic symptom, Ganser's original patients all had clouded consciousness, hallucinations, and somatic conversion symptoms.[12] This uncommon syndrome was originally described in prisoners but is not restricted to this population. It is not typically seen in children. Its etiology is unclear, but some patients have a schizophrenic disorder or an underlying brain disease. The nature and inconsistency of their mental status findings strongly suggest a significant component of either hysteria or malingering. Most patients have some motivating reason to appear legally insane, incompetent, or cognitively impaired.

On occasion, professed memory loss is a conscious and motivated symptom of malingering. It may be associated with other feigned neurologic or psychiatric symptoms but can also be seen alone. The patients whom we have seen usually have a very specific, well-recognized reason for their malingering (in our experience, either avoiding prosecution by virtue of incompetence or gaining compensation for a minor head injury). On examination, these patients may give approximate answers or very bizarre answers. Their memory loss is usually inconsistent, in that they may fail all memory testing but remember a football score from the previous weekend. They also claim patches of remote memory loss and at times claim not to remember their own name.

SUMMARY

In general, memory is a hierarchic process in which information must first be registered in a basic sensory cortical area and then processed through the limbic system for new learning to occur. Finally, the material is permanently established in the appropriate association cortex. At this point, limbic retrieval is no longer required in the recall process. The immediate recall system is disturbed by damage to the primary sensory or motor cortex or by inattention. Learning is prevented by damage to the hippocampi or the dorsal medial thalamic nuclei. Old remote memories are resistant to limbic damage but will be lost when widespread cortical damage occurs. Careful testing of the various aspects of memory can frequently lead to both a clinical and an anatomic diagnosis.

REFERENCES

1. Benson, DF and Geschwind, N: Shrinking retrograde amnesia. J Neurol Neurosurg Psychiatry 30:539, 1967.
2. Benton, A and Spreen, O: Visual memory test performance in mentally deficient and brain-damaged patients. American Journal of Mental Deficiency 68:630, 1964.
3. Bisiach, E and Faglioni, P: Recognition of random shapes by patients with unilateral lesions as a function of complexity, association value, and delay. Cortex 10:101, 1974.
4. Black, FW and Strub, RL: Digit repetition performance in patients with focal brain damage. Cortex 14:12, 1978.
5. Bremner, JD, et al: Deficits in short-term memory in posttraumatic stress disorder. Am J Psychiatry 150:1015–1019, 1993.
6. Breslow, R, Kocsis, J, and Belkin, B: Contribution of the depressive perspective to memory function in depression. Am J Psychiatry 138:227, 1981.
7. DeJong, R, Itabashi, HI, and Olson, J: Memory loss due to hippocampal lesions. Arch Neurol 20:339, 1969.
8. DeJong, R: The hippocampus and its role in memory. J Neurol Sci 19:73, 1973.
9. DeRenzi, E: Nonverbal memory and hemispheric side of lesion. Neuropsychologia 6:181, 1968.
10. Duffy, CJ: Implicit memory: Knowledge without awareness. Neurology 49:1200–1202, 1997.
11. Folstein, MF and McHugh, PP: Dementia syndrome of depression. In Katzman, R, Terry, RD, and Beck, KL (eds): Alzheimer's Disease: Senile Dementia and Related Disorders. Vol 7, Aging. Raven Press, New York, 1978, pp 87–94.
12. Ganser, SJM: A peculiar hysterical state. In Hirsch, SR and Shepherd, M (eds): Themes and Variations in European Psychiatry: An Anthology. J Wright, Bristol, U.K. 1974, pp 67–77.
13. Geschwind, N, Quadfasel, F, and Segarra, J: Isolation of the speech area. Neuropsychologia 67:327, 1968.
14. Heathfield, K, Croft, P, and Swash, M: The syndrome of transient global amnesia. Brain 96:729, 1973.
15. Hodges, JR and Warlow, CP: Syndromes of transient amnesia. J Neurol Neurosurg Psychiatry 53:834, 1990.
16. Kopelman, MD: The Korsakoff syndrome. Br J Psychiatry 166:154–173, 1995.
17. Lewinsohn, P, et al: A comparison between frontal and nonfrontal right and left hemisphere brain-damaged patients. J Comp Physiol Psychol 81:248, 1972.
18. Logan, W and Sherman, DG: Transient global amnesia. Stroke 14:1005, 1983.
19. Markowitsch, J, et al: Retrograde amnesia after traumatic injury of the frontotemporal cortex. J Neurol Neurosurg Psychiatry 56:988–992, 1993.
20. Mathew, N and Meyer, J: Pathogenesis and natural history of transient global amnesia. Stroke 5:303, 1974.

21. Milner, B: Intellectual functions of the temporal lobes. Psychol Bull 51:42, 1954.
22. Natelson, BH, et al: Temporal orientation and education: A direct relationship in normal people. Arch Neurol 36:444, 1979.
23. Neisser, U: Cognitive Psychology. Appleton-Century-Crofts, New York, 1967.
24. Nott, P and Fleminger, J: Presenile dementia: The difficulties of early diagnosis. Acta Psychiatr Scand 51:210, 1975.
25. Parkin, AJ: Residual learning capability in organic amnesia. Cortex 18:417, 1982.
26. Scoville, W and Milner, B: Loss of recent memory after bilateral hippocampal lesions. J Neurol Neurosurg Psychiatry 20:11, 1957.
27. Seeck, M, et al: Neurophysiological correlates of implicit face memory in intracranial visual evoked potentials. Neurology 49:1312–1316, 1997.
28. Selzer, B and Benson, DF: The temporal pattern of retrograde amnesia in Korsakoff's disease. Neurology 24:527, 1974.
29. Simpson, N, Black, FW, and Strub, RL: Memory assessment using the Strub-Black mental status exam and the Wechsler memory scale. J Clin Psychol 42:147, 1986.
30. Smith, A: The Serial Sevens Subtraction Test. Arch Neurol 17:78, 1967.
31. Speedie, LJ and Heilman, KM: Amnestic disturbances following infarction of the left dorsomedial nucleus of the thalamus. Neuropsychologia 20:597, 1982.
32. Speedie, LJ and Heilman, KM: Anterograde memory deficits for visuospatial material after infarction of the right thalamus. Neuropsychologia 40:183, 1983.
33. Squire, LR and Butters, N (eds): Neuropsychology of Memory. The Guilford Press, New York, 1984.
34. Squire, LR and Moore, RY: Dorsal thalamic lesion in a noted case of human memory dysfunction. Ann Neurol 6:503, 1979.
35. Strub, R and Gardner, H: The repetition defect in conduction aphasia: Amnestic or linguistic? Brain Lang 1:241, 1975.
36. Victor, M, Adams, R, and Collins, G: The Wernicke-Korsakoff Syndrome and Related Neurologic Disorders due to Alcoholism and Malnutrition, ed 2. FA Davis, Philadelphia, 1989.
37. Warrington, EK and Weiskrantz, L: Amnesia: A disconnection syndrome. Neuropsychologia 20:233, 1982.
38. Ween, JE, Verfaellie, M, and Alexander, MP: Verbal memory function in mild aphasia. Neurology 47:795–801, 1996.
39. Wilson, R, et al: Primary memory and secondary memory in dementia of the Alzheimer type. J Clin Neuropsychol 5:337, 1983.
40. Zola, S: Amnesia: Neuroanatomic and clinical aspects. In Feinberg, TE and Farah, MJ (eds): Behavioral Neurology and Neuropsychology. McGraw-Hill, New York 1997, pp 447–462.

CONSTRUCTIONAL ABILITY

Constructional ability (constructional praxis or visuoconstructive ability) is the ability to draw or construct two- or three-dimensional figures or shapes. Copying line drawings using pencil on paper, reproducing matchstick patterns, and reconstructing block designs are all examples of routinely used tests of constructional ability. *Such constructional tasks are extremely useful for detecting organic brain disease and should be included in every mental status examination. A high-level, nonverbal cognitive function, constructional ability is a very complex perceptual motor ability involving the integration of occipital, parietal, and frontal lobe functions.* Because of the extensive cortical area necessary to perform constructional tasks, early or subtle brain damage frequently disrupts performance. In some patients, the unsuccessful attempt to copy a simple line drawing can be the only objective evidence suggesting organic brain disease.

Despite their importance and proven clinical use, constructional tasks are not always included in bedside or office mental status testing, partly because very few patients actually complain of constructional impairment. Architects or engineers, whose professions require such abilities, might notice difficulty when drawing plans, reading blueprints, or translating plans into actual construction, but most patients are quite surprised to find that they are unable to draw a clock or copy a block design when asked to do so. Because constructional tests take only a few minutes to perform and can yield very valuable data, we encourage every clinician to use them.

We use the term "constructional ability," rather than the more classic term "constructional praxis," to discuss this general area of cognitive function. "Praxis," in the strict sense, refers to the motor integration used to execute complex learned movements. The reproduction of line drawings or block designs involves more than the organization of skilled hand movements. Such reproduction requires accurate visual perception, integration of perception into kinesthetic images, and translation of kinesthetic images into the final motor patterns that are necessary to produce the construction. Patients do not have to recognize or name the figure; they only have to develop an accurate concept or gestalt. The relations of angles and sides, the integration of parts into a whole, orientation on the page, and three-dimensionality must all be appreciated for accurate motor integration to occur. The final step, of course, requires adequate limb strength and coordination.

We use "constructional impairment," rather than "constructional apraxia," to describe the failure to perform adequately on any of these tasks. As implied in the preceding paragraph, a disturbance in praxis (apraxia) refers only to a breakdown in the execution of the learned movements that are involved in the constructional task.[10] The term "apraxia" excludes the component of visual perception and organization and thus does not accurately describe the neuropsychologic complexity of the entire process.

EVALUATION

As with any skilled motor activity, both initial exposure and repeated practice affect the ability to reproduce paper-and-pencil designs or to complete block constructions. Social deprivation and a lack of academic experience, therefore, have a detrimental effect on constructional performance. The clinician who uses constructional tests as a part of the mental status examination must be cautious in interpreting the results of performance of patients with a history of retardation, a poor academic background, or both. Placed in the proper interpretive context, however, use of drawings and other constructional tests may be productive in such patients.

Selecting Tests of Constructional Ability

Constructional ability may be tested in a variety of ways, and *different levels of performance may be found in the same patient when different tests are employed.* To show the range of test materials that may be used, Warrington[25] has listed six basic types of tests for eliciting evidence of constructional impairment:

- Two-dimensional block designs
- Paper-and-pencil reproduction of geometric shapes
- Spontaneous drawings
- Stick-pattern reproduction
- Three-dimensional block constructions
- Spatial analysis tasks that require the patient to shade in the portion of a design that is common to two or more overlapping figures

Patients with brain lesions show differences in the incidence, severity, and quality of constructional impairment, depending on the type of test used and the nature, size, and location of their lesions.[1,3,22] The clinical examination of constructional impairment in each patient ideally should include several tests to tap somewhat different aspects of constructional ability; however, reproduction drawings and drawings to command are the easiest tests to administer and interpret.

The use of the tests outlined in this book presumes that the patient has adequate visual acuity (at least 20/100, as objectively tested) and sufficient motor ability to use paper, pencil, and blocks effectively. Deficits in either motor or sensory channels can hinder performance, but such impairment does not reflect the disruption in the integrative higher cortical function that these tests are designed to assess.

Several constructional tests that include a memory component are available.[4,11,21] Although the inclusion of the memory component does increase the sensitivity of constructional tests, it also raises serious problems in the interpretation of the test results. Deficits in drawings from memory may be due to memory problems, constructional problems, or a combination of the two. We believe that memory is an important enough variable to warrant testing it specifically in isolation. As we have emphasized throughout this book, *a primary goal of each aspect of mental status testing is to assess each cognitive function as discretely as possible.* The reader is referred to Appendix 1 for further information regarding the availability and description of visual memory tests.

The following brief tests of constructional ability are included for bedside and office testing. *These tests were chosen because of their ease of administration and interpretation, their limited need for apparatus and specialized equipment, and their proven efficacy in the detection of diffuse and focal brain lesions in patients with a wide range of intelligence.*[24]

Reproduction Drawings

We suggest that reproduction drawings be administered first when assessing constructional ability because of their apparent simplicity and familiarity.

DIRECTIONS: The drawings presented in Figure 7–1 can be reproduced adequately by normal individuals and are very sensitive to the effects of brain disease. They are organized in order of increasing difficulty and should be so administered. Both two- and three-dimensional drawings are used because of frequent quantitative and qualitative performance differences noted on these two somewhat different tasks. The examiner either may use a standard predrawn set of designs (probably best because the stimuli are identical for each administration and are generally of better quality than quickly drawn bedside examples) or may draw the stimulus figures on the left side of a piece of blank white paper. It is helpful to use two colors of pencil or felt-tip pen, to reduce the possibility of confusion between the drawings of the patient and those drawn by a hurried examiner. Separate sheets of paper for each design

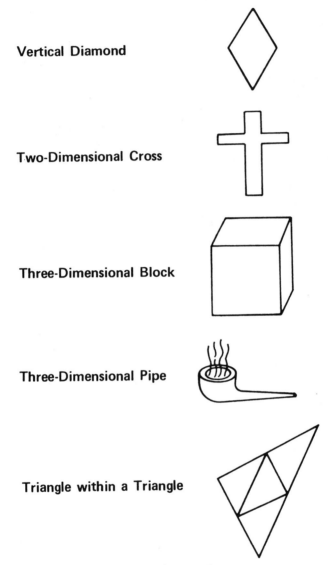

Vertical Diamond

Two-Dimensional Cross

Three-Dimensional Block

Three-Dimensional Pipe

Triangle within a Triangle

FIGURE 7–1. Test items for Reproduction Drawings Test.

may be needed for patients who are highly distractible or perseverative. Lined progress-note forms, consult sheets, and other handy paper that is perceptually confusing should not be used. Patients who become frustrated with their efforts on one drawing should be encouraged by the examiner either to start over or to go on to the next drawing.

Introduce each item by saying, "Please draw this design exactly as it looks to you" (see Fig. 7–1).

SCORING: To help the examiner quantify the adequacy of patients' performance on this test, an objective scoring system[18] is provided for rating the relative quality of each drawing.

0—Poor	Given for nonrecognizable reproductions or a gross distortion of the basic design gestalt
1—Fair	Given for moderately distorted or rotated two-dimensional drawings or a loss of all three-dimensionality with moderate distortions or rotations on three-dimensional designs
2—Good	Given for minimal distortions or rotations with adequate integration on two-dimensional designs and some evidence of three-dimensionality but less-than-perfect reproduction on three-dimensional designs
3—Excellent	Given for perfect (or nearly perfect) reproductions of two- and three-dimensional drawings

As illustrated in Figure 7–2, drawings that show evidence of rotations of more than 90 degrees, perseveration, or "closing in" are given ratings of 0.

Standardization of these designs comparing their use with nonselected brain-damaged individuals and with low-IQ (less than 80) normal people has indicated highly significant ($P < .0001$) differences in performance by the two groups on each design. A rating of 0 on any design resulted in a 100% probability of the patient being correctly classified as brain-damaged, with a 0% probability of misclassification (false-positive). A rating of 1 resulted in an 80% probability of brain damage.[24]

Although the clinician soon gains familiarity with this test and develops his or her own scoring criteria based on experience, examples from our clinical population representing poor, fair, good, and excellent drawing reproductions are shown in Figures 7–3 through 7–7 to help the examiner rate each design.

Drawings to Command

DIRECTIONS: The patient is required to draw three pictures, according to verbal commands. Introduce the test by saying, "I would now like you to draw some simple pictures on this paper. Draw each picture as well as you are able. Please draw a picture of a clock with the numbers and hands on it; a daisy in a flowerpot; and a house in perspective, so that you can see two sides and the roof."

SCORING: A simple scoring system similar to that used with reproduction drawings may be used to aid the examiner in quantifying performance on this test.

Example 1 ROTATION

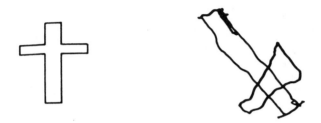

Example 2 PERSEVERATION

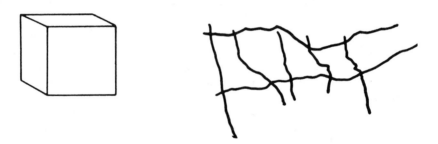

Example 3 "Closing In"

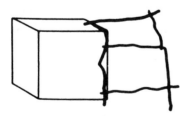

FIGURE 7–2. Examples of patient drawings with specific types of errors.

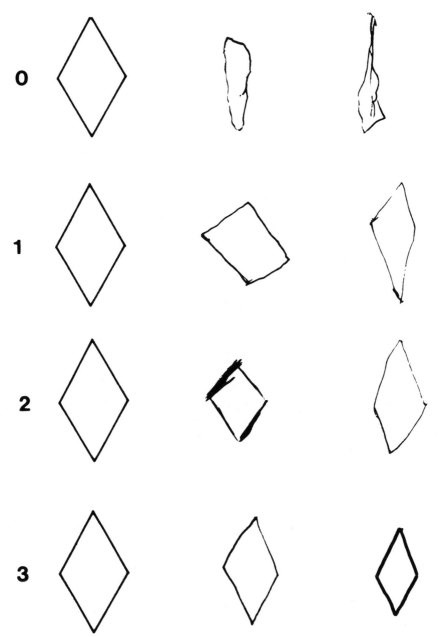

FIGURE 7-3. Renderings of Vertical Diamond Test, with scores of 0 (poor) through 3 (excellent).

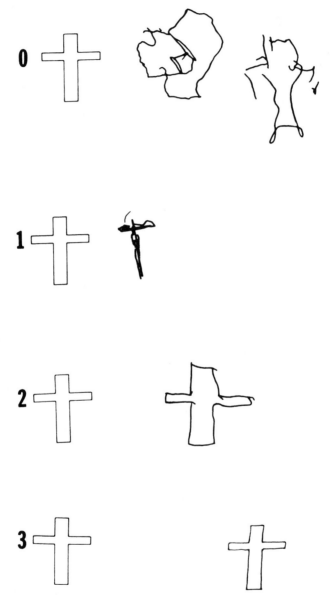

FIGURE 7 – 4. Renderings of Two-Dimensional Cross Test, with scores of 0 (poor) through 3 (excellent).

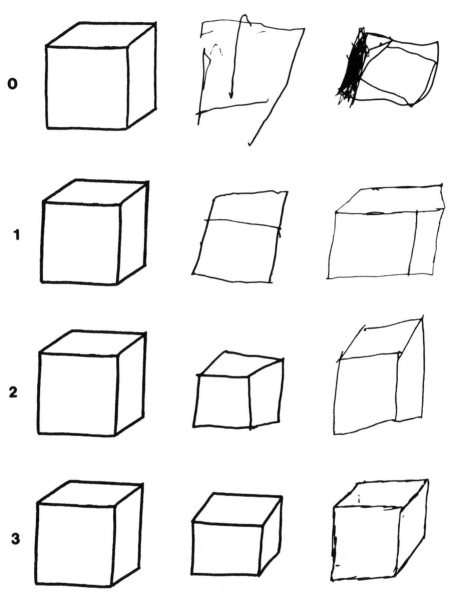

FIGURE 7–5. Renderings of Three-Dimensional Cube Test, with scores of 0 (poor) through 3 (excellent).

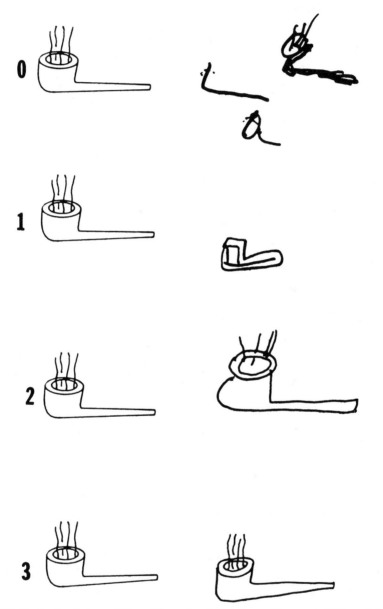

FIGURE 7 – 6. Renderings of Three-Dimensional Pipe Test, with scores of 0 (poor) through 3 (excellent).

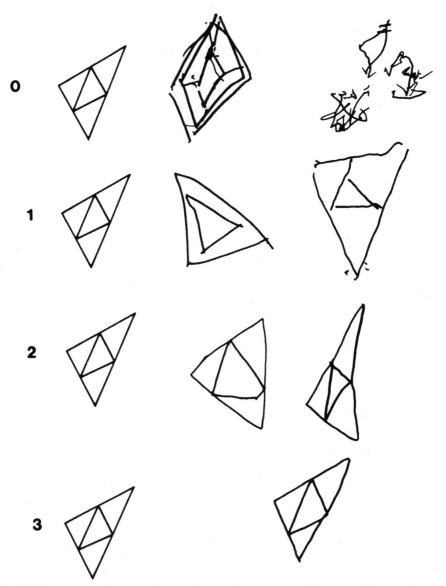

FIGURE 7 – 7. Renderings of Triangle Within a Triangle Test, with scores of 0 (poor) through 3 (excellent).

0—Poor	Given for nonrecognizable drawings or a gross distortion of the basic gestalt
1—Fair	Given for moderate distortion or rotation of any of the drawings or a loss of three-dimensionality on the house drawing (the clock should contain an approximately circular face or the numbers 1 through 12; the daisy should be recognizable as a flower in a pot; and the house should be recognizable as a house)
2—Good	Given for only mild distortions with adequate integration on all pictures (the house should contain some evidence of three-dimensionality and contain the basic elements of a house; the clock should contain two of the following: circular face, numbers 1 through 12, and symmetric number placement; the daisy should be in the generally appropriate shape—a circular center with petals around it)
3—Excellent	Given for perfect (or near perfect) representations of the items with all appropriate components, placement, and perspective (the house and flowerpot should be clearly three-dimensional)

Representative clinical examples of poor, fair, good, and excellent drawings are shown in Figures 7–8 through 7–10, to help the examiner rate each picture.

The clock setting task can often bring out interesting errors, not only in pure constructional ability but also in the conceptualization of time and its abstract relation to the placement of the hands. Many patients with early dementia can draw the clock and put in the numbers correctly, but when asked to set the hands at 2:30, they will ponder, then put one hand on 2 and the other on 3 and add a 0, or put in three hands (one on the 12, one on the 3, and one on the 6), or draw a straight line from the 2 to the 6 (Fig. 7–11). Freedman and Kaplan[8,14] have studied clock drawings extensively and suggest asking patients to set a time in which one hand is on the left side of the clock face and one on the right (e.g., 11:10 or 10:20) in order to identify errors that might arise if a patient has unilateral neglect. In their studies, patients over age 70 made increasingly frequent errors in clock setting.

Block Designs

The following test, although important and often a source of excellent clinical data, does require equipment other than paper and pencil and is therefore considered ancillary.

DIRECTIONS: The use of this test requires four multicolored cubes (obtained from the suppliers of the Wechsler's Adult Intelligence Scale [WAIS-R or WAIS-III] or from many toy stores as Kohs blocks) and four stimulus designs, which may be drawn with colored pens or pencils on pieces of heavy white paper. The stimulus designs should be accurately drawn in the approximate size of the design completed with blocks. The designs in Figure 7–12 are arranged in ascending order of difficulty. Take four blocks and say, "These blocks are all alike. On some sides they are all red; on some, all white; and on some half red and half white. I would like you to take these blocks and

0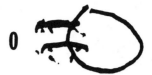

1

2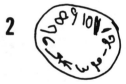

3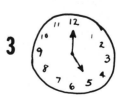

FIGURE 7–8. Renderings of Drawings to Command Test (clock), with scores of 0 (poor) through 3 (excellent).

0

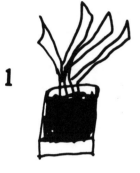

1

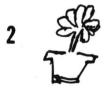

2

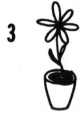

3

FIGURE 7-9. Renderings of Drawings to Command Test (flowerpot), with scores of 0 (poor) through 3 (excellent).

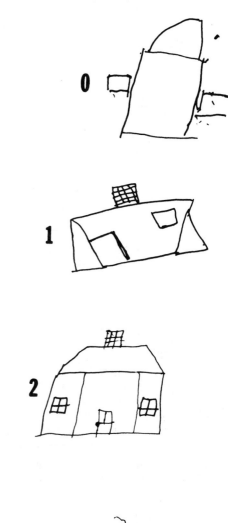

FIGURE 7–10. Renderings of Drawings to Command Test (house in perspective), with scores of 0 (poor) through 3 (excellent).

DRAW A CLOCK FACE
    WITH ALL NUMBERS.

SET CLOCK FOR
    2:30.

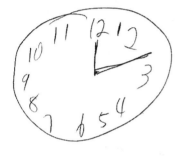

FIGURE 7–11. Common errors seen on clock-setting task.

make a design (or picture) that looks like this picture." If the patient fails to reproduce design 1 accurately, score the response as a failure and demonstrate the correct reproduction. Continue with each design in turn, being sure to mix up the blocks after each effort.

SCORING: Only perfect reproductions of the designs are considered correct. Rotations (either right-left or near-far) are scored as incorrect, as are figure-ground (color) reversals. A score of 1 is given for each correctly reproduced design. Normal individuals are expected to reproduce each design perfectly.

Examples of commonly seen rotation, reversal, and "stringing out" errors are shown in Figure 7–13.

Interpreting Test Performance

Normal individuals obtain almost-perfect scores on simple reproduction and command drawings, but a modest yet significant dropoff in performance oc-

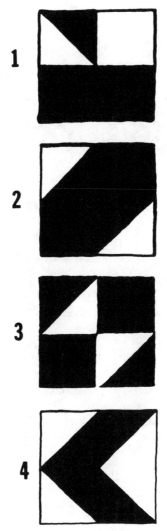

FIGURE 7-12. Test items for Block Designs Test.

curs with increasing age (Table 7-1). The three-dimensional cube and the house are the most difficult. Close inspection of the data in Table 7-1 shows how much overlap exists among normal individuals (particularly the elderly), as well as the considerable overlap between normal elderly and patients with early dementia. *Subtle evidence of constructional impairment, therefore, must be cautiously interpreted.*

Several specific types of errors on constructional tests are usually accepted as almost pathognomonic of brain damage when made by a nonretarded patient over age 10. Most of these errors can be seen on both paper-and-pencil and

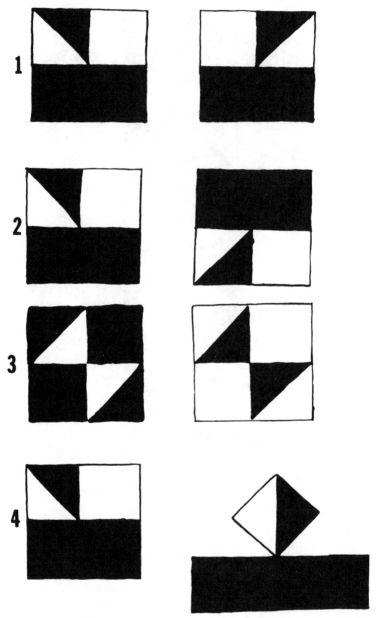

FIGURE 7–13. Common errors seen on Block Designs Test. (1) Right-left rotation. (2) Near-far rotation. (3) Figure-ground reversal. (4) "Stringing out."

TABLE 7 – 1. Construction Performance*

Age	Diamond	Cross	Cube	Pipe	Triangles	Clock	Flower	House
Normal Individuals (by age group)								
40–49	2.8 (0.4)	2.8 (0.4)	2.3 (0.7)	2.6 (0.5)	2.9 (0.4)	2.9 (0.3)	2.6 (0.6)	2.2 (0.7)
50–59	2.9 (0.3)	2.8 (0.4)	2.4 (0.5)	2.6 (0.5)	2.9 (0.4)	3.0 (0.2)	2.7 (0.6)	2.5 (0.5)
60–69	2.7 (0.5)	2.6 (0.5)	2.1 (1.0)	2.5 (0.7)	2.7 (0.5)	2.5 (0.7)	2.5 (0.7)	2.2 (0.7)
70–79	2.6 (0.5)	2.2 (0.5)	1.6 (0.7)	2.1 (0.7)	2.5 (0.8)	2.3 (0.7)	2.2 (0.7)	2.1 (0.7)
80–89	2.8 (0.4)	2.2 (0.6)	1.9 (1.0)	2.0 (0.8)	2.5 (0.5)	2.1 (0.9)	1.9 (0.9)	1.9 (0.8)
Patients with Alzheimer's Disease (by stage and age)								
I (age 71.3 ± 7.8)	2.5 (0.5)	2.2 (0.9)	2.0 (0.7)	2.2 (0.5)	2.4 (0.6)	2.7 (0.5)	1.9 (0.9)	1.8 (0.9)
II (age 71.6 ± 7.1)	2.4 (0.7)	1.9 (0.8)	1.6 (0.9)	1.8 (0.7)	2.0 (0.9)	1.8 (1.0)	1.5 (0.8)	1.4 (0.9)
III (age 71.5 ± 8.9)	1.5 (1.1)	1.2 (1.0)	0.9 (0.9)	0.9 (0.8)	1.1 (1.0)	0.6 (0.9)	0.5 (0.6)	0.5 (0.8)

*Mean (SD), on a scale of 0 to 3.

block-design tests. The most important of these pathognomonic signs are the following:

1. Rotation by more than 45 degrees or the disorientation of the whole figure or a component of it on the background
2. Perseveration or the repetition of the entire figure or part of it
3. Fragmentation of the design or the omission of parts of the figure
4. Significant difficulty in either integration or the placement of individual parts at the correct angles or location
5. Substitution or addition of "dog-ears" for angles on the drawn figure.

Any of these errors should raise a strong question of brain dysfunction requiring more detailed evaluation.

ANATOMY

The parietal lobes are the principal cortical areas involved in visual-motor integration. The visual receptive areas of the occipital lobes and the motor areas of the frontal lobes are necessary for the completion of all of the tests, but it is the association cortex of the parietal lobes that is responsible for most of the complex integration. The actual localization of the various aspects of construction within the parietal lobes is not established, but visual stimuli are thought to spread from primary sensory area 17 to contiguous secondary association areas of the inferior parietal lobule (areas 39 and 40), where associations are made among visual, auditory, and kinesthetic images.[19] Kinesthetic analysis of the visual pattern is the initial task of the association area. The kinesthetic images are then translated into motor patterns by involving the perirolandic premotor area. Drawings to command also require input from the auditory system. The premotor frontal association cortex would theoretically seem to be very important in these highly skilled, fine motor tasks, but, in fact, only a small percentage of patients with lesions restricted to the frontal lobes have constructional impairment.[7] The parietal lobes seem to be the major areas involved in learning and programming skilled movements; the frontal motor areas appear to be more involved in the pure executive nature of the task. (A more extensive discussion of deficits in learned skilled movements is in the section on apraxia in Chapter 9.)

CLINICAL IMPLICATIONS
Locating Lesions

If a nonretarded adult demonstrates constructional impairment on the tests outlined in this chapter, parietal lobe dysfunction should be strongly suspected. Although lesions in any quadrant of the brain can disrupt constructional performance, the incidence and severity of the deficits in patients with lesions restricted to the frontal lobes are small. Most constructional impairment is seen in patients with cortical damage posterior to the rolandic fissure.[7,15]

It was once believed that the right (nondominant) parietal lobe was actually dominant for constructional ability. Many studies have been performed comparing the relative incidence and severity of constructional impairment in patients with lesions of the right and left hemispheres. These studies clearly demonstrate that performance can be defective with lesions in either parietal lobe.[20] *In general, right hemisphere lesions produce a higher incidence and greater severity of defect than do left hemisphere lesions.*[3] What is certain is that constructional ability is not a function exclusive to the right parietal lobe.[12]

Some subtle differences in qualitative performance that are both interesting and possibly useful in clinical testing have been noted in patients with right and left parietal lobe lesions. On the block designs test, patients with right hemisphere lesions frequently lose the basic outline of the design and "string out" the blocks[13] (example 4, see Fig. 7–13). These patients tend to make scattered and fragmented drawings that show loss of spatial relations and orientation on the page. Patients with left hemisphere lesions show more coherent block designs, with maintenance of external configuration but loss of accurate internal detail (example 3, see Fig. 7–13). Their drawings tend to be simplifications of the model, lacking detail but having preserved general spatial relationships. Obvious differences in the performance of the two groups are not always seen, and elaborate scoring schemes have been designed to bring out the subtle differences.[5] Such systems are interesting but are probably not of practical significance to the bedside clinician. The quality of constructional impairment with right hemisphere lesions is uniform and will not differ according to the locus of the lesion within the hemisphere.[16] Without very careful assessment of qualitative performance and using constructional tests alone, it is not always possible to determine the side of the lesion in the individual patient unless unilateral neglect is present. When a patient with normal language shows grossly impaired constructional ability, right hemisphere dysfunction is strongly suggested.

Patients with lesions confined to the parietal lobes often show evidence of significant constructional impairment on mental status testing but fail to demonstrate abnormalities on the standard neurologic examination. Therefore, *the presence of errors on constructional ability testing should lead to a more complete neurodiagnostic workup.*

Identifying Cortical Disease

The most dramatic examples of constructional impairment occur in patients with bilateral cortical disease, particularly cerebral atrophy. Patients with Alzheimer's disease (by far the most common dementia) may show constructional difficulty in the early stages of their disease (see Table 7–1).[23] Patients with multiple infarct dementia, seen in cerebral vascular disease, may also demonstrate constructional impairment, but they usually have other abnormal neurologic signs as well. Patients in confusional states from toxic or metabolic factors frequently demonstrate constructional impairment during the acute stage. This is secondary to reversible physiologic disturbance of the cortex rather than to structural damage.

Because of the fairly high incidence of constructional impairment in dementia, such tasks are very good screening tests in patients of advancing age who present with vague psychiatric or neurologic complaints.

Evaluating Maturation

Standard drawing and other constructional ability tests are used not only to detect brain disease, but also by psychologists to evaluate both the maturational stage of perceptual motor development (constructional ability) and the presence of specific constructional problems in children. The ability to integrate visual stimuli and to construct or draw a reproduction is closely related to both chronologic and intellectual maturation in young children.[2,9,18] Errors in construction, including poor integration of the parts, distortions or simplification, perseveration, and rotations, are common early in development (age 5 to 7) and tend to decrease with age.[6] Relatively errorless performance on simple drawing tests is expected by age 10 to 12.[18] Measured intelligence tends to be relatively highly correlated with constructional performance in children; for adults of normal intelligence (i.e., IQ above 85) IQ appears to have a limited effect on constructional ability.[21] Both children and adults with a significant mental deficiency tend to show inferior performance on most constructional tests.[4] Formal studies have indicated that it is difficult but not impossible to use drawing tests to differentiate intellectually impaired (e.g., IQ below 70) but socially and vocationally independent adults from similar individuals with demonstrable brain damage.[24]

SUMMARY

Constructional ability is a highly developed cortical integrative function that is primarily carried out in the parietal lobes. Drawings and block constructions are easily administered tests to evaluate this function. Constructional impairment usually suggests disease of the posterior portions of the cerebral hemispheres, although other areas of the cortex may be involved. Because constructional ability is so frequently disturbed in patients with brain disease, testing this function is a very important and highly useful component of the mental status examination.

REFERENCES

1. Arrigoni, G and DeRenzi, E: Constructional apraxia and hemispheric locus of lesions. Cortex 1:170, 1964.
2. Bender, L: A Visual Motor Gestalt Test and its Clinical use. American Orthopsychiatric Association, New York, 1983.

3. Benson, DF and Barton, M: Disturbances in constructional ability. Cortex 6:19, 1970.
4. Benton, A: Revised Visual Retention Test. The Psychological Corporation, New York, 1974.
5. Benton, AL: Visuoperceptive, visuospatial and visuoconstructive disorders. In Heilman, KM and Valenstein, E (eds): Clinical Neuropsychology, ed 3. Oxford University Press, New York, 1993, pp 165–213.
6. Black, FW: Reversal and rotation errors by normal and retarded readers. Percept Mot Skills 36:895, 1973.
7. Black, FW and Strub, RL: Constructional apraxia in patients with discrete missile wounds of the brain. Cortex 12:212, 1976.
8. Freedman, M, et al: Clock Drawing: A Neuropsychological Analysis. New York, Oxford University Press, 1994.
9. Frostig, M, Lefever, D, and Whittlesey, J: A developmental test of visual perception for evaluating normal and neurologically handicapped children. Percept Mot Skills 12:383, 1961.
10. Geschwind, N: The apraxias: Neural mechanisms of disorders of learned movement. Am Sci 63:188, 1975.
11. Graham, F and Kendall, B: Memory for Designs Test. Psychology Test Specialists, Missoula, MT, 1960.
12. Hecaen, H: Apraxias. In Filskov, SB and Boll, TJ (eds): Handbook of Clinical Neuropsychology. John Wiley & Sons, New York, 1981, pp 267–286.
13. Kaplan, E: Personal communication, 1973.
14. Kaplan, E: A process approach to neuropsychological assessment. In Bull, T and Bryant, BK (eds): Clinical Neuropsychology and Brain Function: Research Measurement and Practice. American Psychological Association, Washington, DC, 1988, pp 129–167.
15. Kertesz, A: Right hemisphere lesions in constructional apraxia and visuospatial deficit. In Kertesz, A (ed): Localization in Neuropsychology. Academic Press, New York, 1983, pp 455–570.
16. Kertesz, A and Dobrowski, S: Right hemisphere deficits, lesion size and location. J Clin Neuropsychol 3:283, 1981.
17. Kirk, A and Kertesz, A: Subcortical contributions to drawing. Brain Cognition 21:57–70, 1993.
18. Koppitz, E: The Bender Gestalt Test for Young Children. Grune & Stratton, New York, 1964.
19. Luria, A: The Working Brain. Basic Books, New York, 1973.
20. Mack, JL and Levine, RN: The basis of visual constructional disability in patients with unilateral cerebral lesions. Cortex 17:515, 1981.
21. Pascal, G and Suttell, B: The Bender Gestalt Test. Grune & Stratton, New York, 1951.
22. Piercy, M, Hecaen, H, and DeAjuriaguerra, J: Constructional apraxia associated with unilateral lesions: Left and right cases compared. Brain 83:232, 1960.
23. Sjorgen, T, Sjorgen, T, and Lindgren, AGH: Morbus Alzheimer and Morbus Pick: A genetic, clinical, and pathoanatomical study. Acta Psychiatr Scand (Suppl)82:1, 1952.
24. Strub, RL, Black, FW, and Leventhal, B: The clinical utility of reproduction drawings with low IQ patients. J Clin Psychiatry 40:386, 1979.
25. Warrington, E: Constructional apraxia. In Vinken, P and Bruyn, G (eds): Handbook of Clinical Neurology, Vol 4, Disorders of Speech, Perception and Symbolic Behavior. American Elsevier, Amsterdam, 1969, pp 67–83.

CHAPTER

8

HIGHER COGNITIVE FUNCTIONS

Attention, language, and memory are the basic processes that serve as building blocks for the development of higher intellectual abilities. These basic functions are necessary, but not sufficient in and of themselves, to execute more complex cognitive functions. *The higher cognitive functions, including the manipulation of well-learned material, abstract thinking, problem-solving, judgment, arithmetic computations, and so forth, represent the highest level of human intellectual functioning readily assessable by formal testing methods.* These complex neuropsychologic functions are predicated on the integrity and interaction of more basic processes.

Because they represent the most advanced stages of intellectual development, the higher cognitive functions are often highly susceptible to the effects of neurologic disease. The evaluation of these functions in the mental status examination may often demonstrate the early effects of cortical damage before the more basic processes of attention, language, and memory are impaired. *The ability to perform effectively within the environment is determined in large part by an individual's adequacy in performing such higher-order functions.* An assessment of the patient's performance in these areas provides useful diagnostic information, as well as information concerning social and vocational prognosis. The higher cognitive functions are evaluated initially during the history taking, when the patient and others are asked about the patient's adequacy in job performance, management of personal finances, ability to solve problems, and overall judgment.

EVALUATION

The higher cognitive functions may be formally evaluated in many different ways. Most tests of intelligence and higher-order reasoning are based largely on assessments of these functions. In general, *the higher cognitive functions may be categorized in the following hierarchic groupings:*

1. The *fund of acquired information* or the store of knowledge

2. The *manipulation of old knowledge* (e.g., calculations or problem solving)

3. *Social awareness and judgment*

4. *Abstract thinking* (e.g., interpretation of proverbs or the completion of a conceptual series)

The store of basic acquired information is most efficiently assessed by simple verbal tests of vocabulary, general information, and comprehension. Specific examples of these kinds of tests may be seen on any basic intelligence test (e.g., Wechsler's Adult Intelligence Scale—Third Edition [WAIS-III] Vocabulary, Information, Picture Completion). General intelligence, education, and social exposure are closely related to performance on these tasks, and the results of any evaluation must be interpreted in light of this background information.

The manipulation of old knowledge is a more active process, which requires both an intact fund of general information and the ability to apply this information to new or unfamiliar situations. Questions concerning social comprehension and calculation ability may be used to assess this function.

Abstract thinking, which is perhaps the highest level of cognition, may be readily assessed by the use of proverbs, conceptual series, or analogy interpretation.

The following tests are recommended to evaluate a spectrum of relevant higher cognitive functions.

Fund of Information

DIRECTIONS: The questions asked in this test provide a reasonable estimate of the patient's store of knowledge or fund of general information. They are presented in order of increasing difficulty and should be so administered. Continue to ask questions until the test is completed or until the patient has failed three successive questions. If the patient's response is unclear, ask him or her to explain more fully. The examiner may repeat the question if necessary but should not paraphrase the question or spell or explain words that are unfamiliar to the patient.

TEST ITEMS

Questions	Acceptable Responses
1. How many weeks are in a year?	52
2. Why do people have lungs?	To transfer oxygen from air to blood; to breathe
3. Name four people who have been president of the United States since 1940.	Any appropriate presidents
4. Where is Denmark?	Scandinavia, Northern Europe
5. How far is it from New York to Los Angeles?	Any answer between 2300 and 3000 miles
6. Why are light-colored clothes cooler in summer than dark-colored clothes?	Light-colored clothes reflect heat from the sun whereas dark-colored clothes absorb heat
7. What is the capital of Spain?	Madrid
8. What causes rust?	Oxidation: a chemical reaction of metal, oxygen, and moisture
9. Who wrote the Odyssey?	Homer
10. What is the Acropolis?	Site of the Parthenon in Athens, Greece; ancient city on a hill in Athens

SCORING: The patient's answer must either be exact or very closely approximate the acceptable response. In our experience, the average patient with an adequate educational background should answer a minimum of six questions appropriately (Table 8–1). Less adequate performance indicates an impaired fund of general information and suggests reduced intelligence, limited social and educational exposure, or significant dementia. Conversely, more

TABLE 8-1. **Fund of Information Test***

Normal Individuals

Age Group	Mean Score (standard deviation)
40–49	6.7 (2.5)
50–59	6.8 (1.9)
60–69	6.5 (2.0)
70–79	6.3 (2.0)
80–89	5.2 (1.5)

Patients with Alzheimer's Disease

Stage	Mean Score (standard deviation)
I	3.5 (3.9)
II	2.0 (2.9)
III	0.6 (1.1)
IV	0 (0)

*Mean number correct ($\pm$SD)

adequate performance suggests above-average intelligence and education. The fund of information is quite stable over a wide age range; only in the 80s does one find a small yet statistically significant dropoff in this function. By contrast, patients with Alzheimer's disease, even those with mild disease, score only an average of 3.5 of a possible 10 on this task.

Calculations

DIRECTIONS: Calculations are complex neuropsychologic functions that involve the somewhat distinct components of number sense and manipulation. Components of calculations include the following:

Rote tables (e.g., addition, subtraction, and multiplication)
The basic arithmetic concept of carrying and borrowing
Recognition of the signs $(+, -, \times, \div)$
Correct spatial alignment for written calculations[12]

Because these components of calculations may be disturbed in isolation, they are assessed separately. There are many ways of testing the basic concept of numbers (written and verbal) as well as the actual manipulation of the numbers. We have chosen the following items for their overall ease of administration and clinical validity. When evaluating calculations, it is important to require the patient to actually calculate and not merely to recite rote tables (e.g., $4 + 4 = 8$ or $3 \times 5 = 15$). This allows the observation of many different types of errors and provides additional clinical data that are important for describing the nature of the deficit and providing neuroanatomic implications. Performance on calculation is, of course, closely related to educational experience. Tell the patient, "We are now going to do some arithmetic examples. Some will be familiar to you and some will not. Try your best on each one."

Verbal Rote Examples

Read each example in a clear voice in the following form: "What is 4 plus 6?" Record the patient's response.

1. Addition

$4 + 6 = (10)$
$7 + 9 = (16)$

2. Subtraction

$8 - 5 = (3)$
$17 - 9 = (8)$

3. Multiplication

$2 \times 8 = (16)$
$9 \times 7 = (63)$

4. Division

$$9 \div 3 = (3)$$
$$56 \div 8 = (7)$$

Verbal Complex Examples

Read each example in the following form only once: "What is 8 plus 13?" Allow only 20 seconds for a response; a failure to respond within that time, even if a correct response is ultimately given, is scored as a failure. Record the patient's response.

1. Addition

$$14 + 17 = (31)$$

2. Subtraction

$$43 - 38 = (5)$$

3. Multiplication

$$21 \times 5 = (105)$$

4. Division

$$128 \div 8 = (16)$$

Written Complex Examples

Provide the patient with the following written examples. If the patient is inattentive and distractible, it is useful to provide each example on individual cards or to write each new example after the patient completes the previous example. Examples written on a single sheet of paper should be widely separated. Allow a reasonable amount of time for completion of each example. Failure to complete the example within 30 seconds should be noted. Record the patient's response, including errors in alignment.

1. Addition

$$\begin{array}{r} 108 \\ + 79 \\ \hline \end{array}$$

2. Subtraction

$$\begin{array}{r} 605 \\ - 86 \\ \hline \end{array}$$

3. Multiplication

$$\begin{array}{r} 108 \\ \times 36 \\ \hline \end{array}$$

4. Division

$$43\overline{)559}$$

SCORING: Each response should be scored as correct or incorrect. By comparing performance on each computation subtest, the patient's overall level

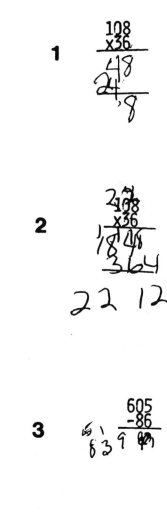

FIGURE 8-1. Examples of calculation errors. (1) Patient with a large right hemisphere lesion and left neglect. (2) Patient with head trauma and a right parietal hematoma. Note poor alignment, as well as other calculation errors. (3) Patient with 2 years of college education, now showing signs of early dementia. (4) Patient with Alzheimer's disease. Note that rote multiplication is good, but basic arithmetic processes have gross problems.

Age Group	Verbal Rote	Verbal Complex	Written
TABLE 8–2. **Tests of Calculation Ability***			
	Normal Individuals (by age group)		
40–49	3.7 (0.7)	2.9 (1.3)	3.4 (1.3)
50–59	3.7 (0.6)	3.1 (0.9)	3.2 (1.1)
60–69	3.7 (0.7)	3.2 (0.8)	3.4 (0.6)
70–79	3.4 (1.0)	2.4 (1.3)	2.8 (1.3)
80–89	3.7 (0.5)	2.9 (1.4)	3.2 (0.8)
	Patients with Alzheimer's Disease (by stage)		
I	3.6 (0.6)	2.9 (1.3)	2.7 (1.0)
II	3.1 (1.0)	1.2 (1.3)	1.9 (1.2)
III	1.6 (1.6)	0.3 (0.8)	0.4 (0.8)
IV	0 (0)	0 (0)	0 (0)

*Mean (SD), on a scale of 0 to 3.

of calculation ability and area of adequacy and deficit can be determined (e.g., intact rote tables, with inability to complete complex, verbally presented examples). Errors specific to a particular aspect of computation (e.g., division) or to a modality of presentation (e.g., intact performance on verbally presented items and impaired performance on written examples) should be noted. Errors involving borrowing and alignment on written examples should be recorded (Fig. 8–1). If an objective measure of arithmetic is needed, the examiner should refer to a standard achievement test such as the Wide Range Achievement Test, Third Edition.[11] Calculation ability is stable across all age groups, although variable performance is seen within each group (Table 8–2). Performance in early dementia is not significantly impaired, particularly in older patients. Performance deteriorates dramatically in the second and third stages of the disease.

Proverb Interpretation

Interpreting proverbs accurately requires an intact fund of general information, the ability to apply this knowledge to unfamiliar situations, and the ability to think in the abstract.

DIRECTIONS: The following proverbs are presented in ascending order of difficulty. Tell the patient, "I am going to read you a saying that you may or may not have heard before. Explain in your own words what the saying means." Read each proverb exactly as it is written; do not paraphrase or otherwise explain the proverb. Continue only until the patient fails on two successive proverbs. If the patient's response to the first proverb is concrete (nonabstract), or if he or she is unable to interpret it, the examiner should supply the correct answer and explain that this is the expected type of response.

TEST ITEMS

1. Don't cry over spilled milk.
2. Rome wasn't built in a day.
3. A drowning man will clutch at a straw.
4. A golden hammer can break down an iron door.
5. The hot coal burns; the cold one blackens.

SCORING: The primary scoring criterion for proverb interpretation is the degree of abstraction demonstrated by the patient in explaining the proverb. It is helpful to rate the quality of the patient's response to each proverb. Because the grading of "abstractness" is somewhat subjective, some investigators have questioned the reliability and therefore the validity of this test.[1] If the examiner properly adjusts his or her expectations based on the level of education or intelligence of the patient, proverb interpretation appears quite reliable and valid.[14] To aid in scoring, examples of abstract (2 points); semiabstract (1 point); and concrete (0 points) responses to each proverb follow. The possible total for this section is 10 points.

---

1. Don't cry over spilled milk.

0—Concrete	"The milk's all over the floor."
	"When the milk is on the floor, you can't use it."
1—Semiabstract	"It's gone; don't worry about it."
	"Don't cry when something goes wrong."
2—Abstract	"Once something is over, don't worry about it."
	"Don't be concerned about events that are beyond control."

2. Rome wasn't built in a day.

0—Concrete	"It took a long time to build Rome."
	"You can't build cities overnight."
1—Semiabstract	"Don't do things too fast."
	"You have to be patient and careful."
2—Abstract	"If something is worth doing, it is worth doing it carefully."
	"It takes time to do things well."

3. A drowning man will clutch at a straw.

0—Concrete	"Don't let go when you're in the water."
	"He's trying to save himself."
1—Semiabstract	"Self-preservation is important."
	"It's a last resort."
2—Abstract	"A person in trouble will try anything to get out of it."
	"If sufficiently desperate, a person will try anything."

4. A golden hammer can break down an iron door.

0—Concrete	"Gold can't break iron!"
	"Gold is too soft to break a door."
1—Semiabstract	"Gold's worth more than iron."
	"The harder something is, the more you have to work to get it."
2—Abstract	"Money can get whatever you want."
	"Virtue conquers all."
	"If you have sufficient knowledge, you can accomplish even the most difficult task."

5. The hot coal burns; the cold one blackens.

0—Concrete	"Hot coals will burn you and leave it black."
	"Hot coals get black when they're cold."
1—Semiabstract	"Coal can have many uses."
	"Getting burned and dirty are both bad."
2—Abstract	"Extremes of anything can be detrimental."
	"There may be bad aspects to things that appear good."

Concrete responses are pathologic in all but the retarded or illiterate patient. The average patient should provide abstract interpretations to at least the first three proverbs and minimally semiabstract responses to the remaining proverbs. Often, uneducated patients will initially give a concrete response but can give abstract interpretations when specifically asked if there is another way of explaining the proverb. Such cued responses should be scored as semiabstract responses. A total score of less than 5 on proverb interpretation is suspicious. A concrete response or an absence of any abstract responses should suggest an impairment of abstract ability.

Performance on proverb interpretation is stable across all ages (Table 8–3). The high standard deviation within the normal population, however, shows how cautious the examiner must be in interpreting a low score on this task. Familiarity with the proverb is an additional factor in judging the abstracting ability of the patient.[5] A very familiar saying that the patient has heard all his or her life may not need much verbal reasoning to interpret because it is merely a piece of advice that has been repeatedly applied to a standard situation. The average score of patients with early Alzheimer's disease is only slightly lower than the average for normal individuals. As dementia progresses, performance drops rapidly. In general, a score of

TABLE 8-3. Tests of Verbal Abstraction*		
Age Group	Proverbs	Similarities
Normal Individuals (by age group)		
40–49	5.1 (1.5)	6.0 (2.5)
50–59	5.1 (1.5)	5.9 (1.9)
60–69	4.4 (2.2)	5.0 (2.3)
70–79	4.3 (1.6)	4.5 (2.0)
80–89	5.6 (1.3)	5.1 (2.6)
Patients with Alzheimer's Disease (by stage)		
I	4.0 (2.3)	4.9 (2.1)
II	1.8 (1.5)	2.8 (2.1)
III	0.5 (0.9)	0.9 (1.4)
IV	0 (0)	0 (0)

*Mean (SD), on a scale of 0 to 3.

2 or 3 on proverb interpretation in educated individuals indicates organic impairment.

Similarities

In the **Verbal Similarities Test**, the patient must explain the basic similarity between two overtly different objects or situations. *This test of verbal abstract ability requires analysis of relationships, formation of verbal concepts, and logical thinking.*

    DIRECTIONS: Tell the patient, "I am going to tell you some pairs of objects. Each pair is alike in some way. Please tell me how they are similar, or alike." If the patient mentions a difference between the items, fails to respond, or states that they are different, score the item 0, provide the appropriate response, and continue with the next item. Give no help on succeeding items. The following test items are presented in ascending order of difficulty.

    TEST ITEMS
1. Turnip—Cauliflower
2. Car—Airplane
3. Desk—Bookcase
4. Poem—Novel
5. Horse—Apple

    SCORING: The response for each item pair is scored for adequacy. Two points should be given for any abstract similarity or general classification that is highly pertinent for both items in the pair. One point should be given for responses that indicate specific properties of both items in the pair and that constitute a relevant similarity. A score of 0 is given when the response reflects properties of only one member of the pair, differences or generalizations that are not pertinent to the item pair, and failures to respond. Following are examples of responses receiving 2 points, 1 point, and 0 points. Total for this section is 10 points.

    1. Turnip—Cauliflower

       2 points: Vegetables
       1 point: Food; grow in the ground; edible
       0 points: Buy in the store; one is a root, the other grows above ground

    2. Car—Airplane

       2 points: Modes of transportation
       1 point: Drive them both; both have motors
       0 points: One's in the air and one's on the road

    3. Desk—Bookcase

       2 points: Articles of furniture; office furniture
       1 point: Household objects; put books on them; made of the same material
       0 points: Sit at a desk and put books in the bookcase; for studying

4. Poem—Novel

2 points: Literary works or types of literature; artistic works; modes of creative expression

1 point: Write them both; tell stories; express feelings

0 points: Famous things; study them in school; people like them

5. Horse—Apple

2 points: Living things; God's living objects, organic things

1 point: Both grow; both have skins; both need food

0 points: Horses eat apples; one is big and one is small; we use them

The nonretarded patient with a normal educational background should obtain a score of 5 or 6 on this test (see Table 8–3). Two concrete (0-point) responses or a total score of less than 4 suggests reduced general intelligence or impaired abstract thinking ability. In general, performance on this test should be compatible with performance on the fund of information and proverb interpretation tests. *Equal impairment on this and the fund of information test suggests retardation or educational deprivation rather than a specific deficit in abstract thinking.*

Insight and Judgment

Insight and judgment are other high-level behavioral functions that can be affected by brain disease. These behaviors are different, yet interrelated. *Insight is one's ability to understand either oneself or an external situation. Judgment is a complex mental process whereby a person forms an opinion, makes a decision, or plans an action or response after first analyzing the issue and comparing choices with acceptable social behavior.*

Insight can be assessed by asking patients whether they are aware of their problem, such as memory loss. A high percentage of demented patients do not appreciate the fact that they have a problem, a situation that is protective for the patient yet often frustrating to others. Lack of insight, or denial, is also seen in patients with large right hemisphere lesions.

Assessing judgment is more difficult, as the quality of judgment varies widely in the normal population; what the examiner is attempting to evaluate, therefore, is a *change* in the patient's judgment. Basic social awareness and problem-solving may be evaluated by questions about environmental situations and how to deal with them effectively (e.g., What should a person do if he or she sees smoke or fire in a grocery store?). Social judgment is a more complex function that includes the basic knowledge of social situations, knowledge of the socially appropriate responses in such situations, and the ability to apply the correct responses personally when faced with an actual social situation. Because of the reality-based nature of social judgment, it is difficult to assess validly in an abstract test situation. The patient who, when asked the question in the confines of an office or hospital bed, matter-offactly answers that he or she would calmly inform the store manager of the presence of smoke or fire may act very differently in the actual situation. Therefore, *collaborative data concerning the patient's social judgment are best obtained by history from family members or other informants who have witnessed the patient's actual performance in dealing with day-to-day events.* An alternative possibility, though somewhat cumbersome and inefficient, is to place the patient in actual, but experimental, situations that require an immediate, appropriate social response.

ANATOMY

The higher cognitive functions rely primarily on an intact cerebral cortex, although subcortical lesions can also affect performance. Except for calculating ability, however, these functions have not been well localized in the way that language or constructional ability has. Abstract thinking, the ability to manipulate old knowledge, and similar functions are probably widely represented in the cortex, and subcortical structures are also important in carrying out these highly abstract functions. Because of this diffuse representation, lesions located in various parts of the brain can impair these functions. Impairment is particularly prominent in widespread bilateral disease (e.g., dementia).

Many of these higher cognitive functions are probably localized in the posterior rather than in the frontal areas of the brain. Social judgment is the major exception. Patients who have frontal lesions often show very poor social judgment despite normal cognitive functioning. Although a loss of abstraction has been described in patients following frontal lobectomies[14] and has been traditionally considered a sign of extensive frontal lobe dysfunction, patients with frontal lobe damage also have defects of attention, memory, and perseveration that may well account for the observed deficits in higher cognition.[10,15] In a comprehensive review of the literature concerned with the interaction of frontal lesions and cognitive functioning, Teuber[16] concluded that such lesions generally affect intelligence less than do lesions located in the more posterior areas of the brain. Black[2] also documented the differential effects of frontal and nonfrontal unilateral lesions on cognitive functions, verifying again that these higher cognitive functions are more commonly impaired with posterior lesions.

Verbal reasoning and abstraction are primarily dominant-hemisphere functions having very close relationships with language. Thus, dominant-hemisphere lesions frequently interfere with these high-level verbal manipulations.

Impaired performance on calculations may be seen with brain lesions that are bilateral or unilateral on either side.[7] Lesions in somewhat different areas of the brain may cause different types of impaired calculation ability (dyscalculia).[6] Left hemisphere lesions in the right-handed patient typically result in more severe impairment of calculations than do corresponding lesions of the nondominant hemisphere.[3] Because numbers are similar to words, in that they are symbols representing a concept, it is not surprising that there is a strong association between acalculia and language problems. Alexia and agraphia for numbers, so-called aphasic acalculia, is a common finding in mild aphasia.[12] Some patients, however, are alexic for numbers and signs (i.e., +, −, ×, ÷) but not for words. This type of dyscalculia is a significant component of Gerstmann's syndrome (described in Chapter 9), which is secondary to a dominant parietal lobe lesion. Anarithmetria (inability to understand and carry out the complex manipulations of numbers) is usually seen in left hemisphere lesions or in bilateral disease (e.g., dementia). Specific calculation defects have been ascribed to focal frontal, temporal, parietal, and occipital lesions.[9] Impaired calculating ability is most commonly caused by focal lesions in the parietal lobes. Parietal lobe acalculia is characterized by a loss of the ability to understand the meaning of numbers and numeric concepts (e.g., larger or smaller) and by the inability to align numbers correctly on the page, owing to visual-spatial deficits. The malalignment in complex computations can often be the most striking feature in the dyscalculia seen in patients with right parietal lobe lesions. In addition to the cases with cortical involvement, some patients with purely subcortical lesions (e.g., involving the left caudate nucleus) have shown dyscalculia.[4]

CLINICAL IMPLICATIONS

Deficits in higher cognitive functions are most frequently seen in patients with widespread brain disease of any etiology. These deficits may often be the first sign of deterioration in progressive brain diseases such as Alzheimer's disease. Focal dominant parietal lobe lesions may produce defects in verbally mediated functions and must be considered in the differential diagnosis in any patient presenting with a loss of abstract ability or impaired calculations. As discussed previously, lesions of the frontal lobe typically do not interfere with the fund of knowledge, abstract thinking, and problem solving unless other, more basic deficits are also present (e.g., perseveration or aphasia). Conversely, social awareness and judgment in social situations are often impaired in patients with large frontal lesions.

Significant functional disease, particularly schizophrenia, may also cause impaired abstracting ability. Although the concreteness of the schizophrenic patient is frequently different from that of the patient with organic brain disease, at times the deficits may be indistinguishable.

Because of the close relationship between higher cognitive function and general intelligence, mental retardation from whatever cause will result in impaired performance on these tests. Educational deprivation will similarly result in substandard performance that is not of diagnostic significance. The test of fund of information provides a reasonable estimate of current intellectual functioning, which may be combined with data from the history to furnish this background information.

SUMMARY

Higher cognitive functions are measures of the patient's reasoning and problem-solving abilities. These functions are often impaired early in brain disease and thereby offer an effective measure for detecting brain disease in patients with relatively intact performance in other areas (e.g., language or constructional ability). Any deficits will be reflected in the patient's inability to function effectively within the environment. Thus, an evaluation of these functions will aid in making a valid social and vocational prognosis.

REFERENCES

1. Anderson, NC: Reliability and validity of proverb interpretation to assess mental status. Comp Psychiatry 18:465–472, 1977.
2. Black, W: Cognitive deficits in patients with unilateral war-related frontal lobe lesions. J Clin Psychol 32:366, 1976.
3. Boller, F and Grafman, J: Acalculia: Historical development and current significance. Brain Cognition 2:205, 1983.
4. Corbett, AJ, McCusker, EA, and Davidson, OR: Acalculia following a dominant hemisphere subcortical infarct. Arch Neurol 43:964–966, 1986.
5. Cunningham, DM, Ridley, SE, and Campbell, A: Relationship between proverb familiarity and proverb interpretation: Implications for clinical practice. Psychol Rep 60:895–898, 1987.
6. Ferro, JM and Botello, MAS: Alexia for arithmetical signs. A cause of disturbed calculations. Cortex 16:175, 1980.
7. Critchley, M: The Parietal Lobes. Edward Arnold, London, 1953.
8. Grafman, J and Rickard, T: Acalculia. In Feinberg, TE and Farah, MJ (eds): Behavioral Neurology and Neuropsychology. McGraw-Hill, New York, 1997, pp 219–226.
9. Grewel, F: Acalculias. In Vinken, P and Bruyn, G (eds): Handbook of Clinical Neurology, Vol 4, Disorders of Speech, Perception, and Symbolic Behavior. American Elsevier, New York, 1969, pp 181–194.
10. Hécaen, H and Albert, M: Disorders of mental functioning related to frontal lobe pathology. In Benson, DF and Blumer, D (eds): Psychiatric Aspects of Neurologic Disease. Grune & Stratton, New York, 1975, pp 137–149.
11. Kahn, HJ (ed): Cognitive and Neuropsychological Aspects of Calculation Disorders. Brain Cognition 17:97, 1991 (special issue).
12. Levin, HS, Goldstein, FC, and Spiers, PA: Acalculia. In Heilman, KM and Valenstein, E (eds): Clinical Neuropsychology, ed 3. Oxford University Press, New York, 1993, pp 91–120.
13. Reich, JN: Proverbs and the modern mental status exam. Comp Psychiatry 22:528–531, 1981.
14. Rylander, G: Mental Changes After Excision of Cerebral Tissue. Ejnar Munksgaards Forlag, Copenhagen, 1943.
15. Stuss, DT and Benson, DF: Neuropsychological studies of the frontal lobes. Psychol Monogr 95:1, 1984.
16. Teuber, HL: The riddle of frontal lobe function in man. In Warren, J and Akert, K (eds): The Frontal Granular Cortex and Behavior. McGraw-Hill, New York, 1964, pp 410–444.
17. Wilkinson, GS: Wide Range Achievement Test–3 Administration Manual. Wide Range, Inc., Wilmington, DE, 1993.

RELATED COGNITIVE FUNCTIONS

Several specific disorders of cognitive function have been of great interest to neurologists and neuropsychologists. Most are related to high-level motor and sensory processing. For instance, apraxia is a high-level motor distur-bance, and visual agnosia is a high-level perceptual disturbance. For years these functions were classified, along with aphasia, as higher cortical func-tions, but with the advent of more sophisticated imaging techniques (i.e., computed tomography [CT] and magnetic resonance imaging [MRI]), it has been shown that subcortical lesions can also affect them. Understanding these disorders can help clinicians in cerebral localization. In addition, neurobe-haviorists have considerable research interest in understanding these disor-ders. Because each disorder is relatively discrete, a complete discussion of each disorder is presented, including terminology, evaluation, and clinical implications.

APRAXIA

Apraxia is an acquired disorder of learned, skilled, sequential motor movements that cannot be accounted for by elementary disturbances of strength, coordination, sen-sation, or lack of comprehension or attention.[28] *It is an impairment in selecting and organizing the motor innervations needed to execute an action.*[3] Apraxia is not a low-level motor disturbance but rather a **defect in motor planning**, which involves the integrative steps that precede skilled or learned movements. Al-though this discussion concentrates on acquired apraxia, a developmental form of apraxia has also been described.[22] Different types of apraxia may be present, based on the complexity and nature of the task performed.

A motor disturbance characterized by clumsiness or involuntary grasp reflexes in the limb contralateral to a cortical lesion[15] is called a limb-kinetic apraxia. Because patients with this disturbance have difficulty with basic motor control and display abnormal reflexes, their movements do not meet the classic requirements of a true apraxia.

Ideomotor Apraxia

Ideomotor apraxia is the most common type of apraxia. Patients having this form of apraxia fail to perform previously learned motor acts accurately. Impairment can be seen in buccofacial, upper or lower limb, or truncal musculature. The inability to carry out such commands as "Show me how you blow out a match" or "—drink through a straw" is called **buccofacial apraxia**. Difficulty making certain arm or leg movements such as those involved in flipping a coin, saluting, or kicking a ball is called **limb apraxia**. Difficulty with truncal commands such as "Curtsy," "Swing a baseball bat," or "Stand like a boxer" is called an **apraxia of whole body movements**. This disorder is *not* related to a disturbance in comprehension of the verbal command.

Evaluation

There is a hierarchy of difficulty in performing these ideomotor tasks. The most difficult level requires the patient to perform the action to verbal command (e.g., "Show me how to flip a coin"). This movement must be mimed without the actual coin and in the absence of nonverbal cues from the examiner. If the patient fails at this level, the examiner performs the action and asks the patient to imitate it. Most patients with apraxia find imitation easier than miming the movements on command. If the patient again fails, provide the actual object and again ask the patient to follow the command. Use of the actual object is usually the easiest task for the apraxic patient, and many who fail on verbal command and imitation will succeed with the concrete task using the real object. The presence of the object gives the patient additional visual and proprioceptive cues that facilitate performance. Innumerable possible commands can be used to evaluate praxis. The following tests frequently elicit apraxic movements.

Buccofacial Commands

Commands	*Errors*
"Show me how to—":	
1. "Blow out a match."	Difficulty giving short, controlled exhalation; saying "blow"; inhaling; difficulty maintaining appropriate mouth posture
2. "Protrude your tongue."	Inability to stick out tongue; tongue moving in mouth but tending to push against front teeth and not protruding
3. "Drink through a straw."	Inability to sustain a pucker; blowing instead of drawing through the straw; random mouthing movements

When tested for buccofacial praxis, patients may try to cue themselves by pretending to have the object (match or straw) in their hands. This self-cuing facilitates performance and should be discouraged by gently restraining the patients' hands.

Limb Commands

Commands	Errors
"Show me how to—":	
1. "Salute."	Hand over head; hand waving; improper position of hand
2. "Use a toothbrush."	Failure to show any proper grip; failure to open mouth; grossly missing the mouth; using finger to pick teeth; not allowing adequate distance for shaft of toothbrush; using the finger as a toothbrush
3. "Flip a coin."	Movements miming tossing the coin into the air with an open hand; supinating or pronating the hand as though turning a doorknob; flexing the arm without flipping thumb against finger
4. "Hammer a nail."	Moving hand back and forth horizontally; pounding with fist
5. "Comb your hair."	Using fingers as teeth of comb; smoothing the hair; making inexact hand movements
6. "Snap your fingers."	Extension of fingers with patting movements; tapping of finger on thumb; sliding finger off thumb with insufficient force
7. "Kick a ball."	Stamping foot; pushing foot along floor; moving foot laterally
8. "Crush out a cigarette."	Stamping foot; kicking foot on floor

Although ideomotor apraxia is usually a bilateral phenomenon (i.e., seen in both right and left limbs), occasionally ideomotor apraxia is unilateral. Accordingly, commands should be alternated between left and right limbs. Do not have the patient do the same command sequentially with both hands, because visual self-cuing will improve performance on the second trial.

Whole-Body Commands

Commands	Errors
"Show me how to—":	
1. "Stand like a boxer."	Awkward arm position; hands at side
2. "Swing a baseball bat."	Difficulty in placing both hands together; chopping movements
3. "Bow" (for a man) or "Curtsy" (for a woman)	Any inappropriate truncal movement

Clinical Implications

The ability to perform skilled movements on verbal command is closely associated with the language functions of the dominant hemisphere. Because adequate verbal comprehension is a prerequisite to valid praxis testing, brain area A (Fig.

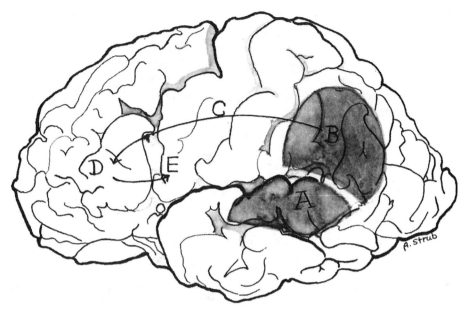

FIGURE 9–1. The pathways for praxis in the right hand (controlled by the left motor area).

9–1) must be intact. Once the command is understood, the information spreads to the contiguous supramarginal gyrus (area B, see Fig. 9–1), where the words (e.g., "flip a coin") are associated with the kinesthetic memories present in the postrolandic parietal cortex. According to the classic model, these sensory memories of the movement are then transferred along pathway C to the premotor area (D), where memory for motor patterns is evoked. The premotor area then directs the pyramidal neurons in the motor strip (E) actually to perform the action. Recent studies have shown that this classic model should be modified, however.[36,53] Information from the parietal area is transferred to the supplementary motor area on the medial frontal lobe (not shown) before going to the motor cortex on the lateral cortex (D&E). A lesion along any of these pathways can cause an ideomotor apraxia. Subcortical structures also have a role in guiding skilled movement, and cases have been described where thalamic lesions, for example, have resulted in severe apraxia.[41] Many patients with lesions in the dominant hemisphere are also aphasic. Accordingly, praxis testing must be very carefully done to ensure that a comprehension deficit is not responsible for the impaired motor performance. Lesions in the areas of the left hemisphere described above can produce a bilateral limb (not buccofacial) apraxia.[53]

The previous paragraph outlined the pathways for praxis in the right hand (controlled by the left motor area). The apraxic patient also has an apraxia with the left hand. Figure 9–2 illustrates that a command to the right

motor cortex for innervation of the left hand is transferred from the left premotor area (D_1) to the right premotor area (D_2) via the anterior callosal fibers
(F_1). Any interruption of this pathway will render the left hand apraxic.[27,28,54]
This is often called a "sympathetic dyspraxia"[26] and can be readily demonstrated in the intact left hand of patients with Broca's aphasia with right
hemiplegia. Lesions of the anterior corpus callosum (F_1) will cause an isolated
apraxia of the left hand; motor and praxis functions of the right hand are
intact.[30] The posterior callosal pathway $(F_2$ to $C_2)$, which could theoretically
transmit the praxis information to the right premotor area (D_2), obviously
does not.

*Lesions of the right hemisphere rarely result in a significant apraxia of either
hand when the patient must carry out the action to command.*[14,19] Some patients
with right hemisphere lesions do, however, have difficulty carrying out actions when asked to imitate the examiner.[3] In such cases the right hemisphere's stronger visual system impairs the patient's perception of the action.

This anatomic model has been verified clinically and pathologically, and

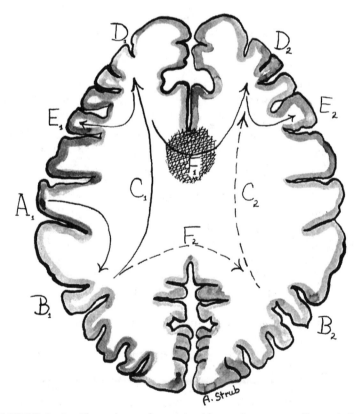

FIGURE 9-2. The pathways for praxis with anterior corpus callosum lesion.

firmly establishes that the hemisphere dominant for language is also dominant for learning skilled movements.[28] This dominance is obvious because most individuals have a strong hand preference for such activities as writing, throwing, and using tools. *Because a lesion of the dominant hemisphere causes an apraxia in both hands, it is apparent that the dominant hemisphere exerts a continual guiding role on movements that originate from the nondominant hemisphere.* Because of the close relationship between language and praxis, many aphasics have an apraxia of the buccofacial musculature. In some patients the apraxia is confined to speech movements, a condition called **verbal apraxia**.

Not all patients with apraxia demonstrate a similar degree and type of impaired performance. Some patients fail completely on command (even when comprehension of the command is adequate), but perform perfectly on imitation. Such patients have a type of disconnection syndrome in which verbal input is literally disconnected from motor areas. Visual input, however, is relayed quickly to the motor areas, and the patient can imitate without difficulty. Most apraxic patients who fail on command, however, also have difficulty with imitation. Some patients have such severe ideomotor apraxia that they fail on verbal command, on imitation, and in the use of actual objects. Some patients with lesions in the left temporoparietal area seem to have considerable difficulty demonstrating the use of simple objects, yet may imitate the action quite well. It has been proposed that this difficulty with real objects is an ideational apraxia rather than a severe ideomotor apraxia and is caused by a memory disorder (of object use) rather than true apraxia.[18] Patients with extensive dominant-hemisphere lesions who cannot carry out movements to command or imitation often show fairly good use of objects such as eating utensils. The performance has some problems in efficiency and organization of movements but is adequate,[23,46] implying that the right hemisphere has sufficient motor engrams for basic tool use.

Whole-body commands can sometimes be performed correctly even in the presence of obvious limb apraxia. They can often be accurately carried out by patients with severe auditory comprehension deficits as well. The reason for the relative sparing of performance involving whole-body commands in some patients is unclear, but it may be due to the fact that these axial movements are under the control of the more widespread extrapyramidal system.[28] As a rule, however, patients with ideomotor limb apraxia also demonstrate apraxic axial movements.[44]

Ideational Apraxia

Classic ideational apraxia is a disturbance of complex motor planning of a higher order than is seen in ideomotor apraxia. It refers to a breakdown in performance of a task that involves a series of related, but separate steps, such as folding a letter, placing it in an envelope, sealing it, and then putting a stamp on it. The patients can often perform each individual step of the task in isolation (e.g.

folding the paper) but cannot integrate the parts accurately to complete the sequence. The patients seem to have lost the overall concept of how to go about completing the task. Some investigators define an ideational apraxia as any difficulty in manipulating real objects.[17,20] We feel that difficulty with object use in simple limb commands (e.g., inability to flip an actual coin) represents a severe ideomotor limb apraxia and not an ideational apraxia. Some patients, however, have for various reasons lost both the concept of the object and its proper use. These individuals are said to exhibit "conceptual apraxia."[43]

Evaluation

Several simple tasks are used to demonstrate an ideational apraxia.

Tasks	Errors
1. Folding a letter, placing it in an envelope, sealing it, addressing it, and placing a stamp on the envelope	Turning paper around without being able to fold it; folding improperly; licking the wrong side of stamp or envelope; inability to place paper in envelope
2. Placing candle in holder, taking match out of box, lighting candle, and blowing out match	Placing candle in holder wick-down; inability to place candle in holder; inability to open or close matchbox; striking match on candle; striking wrong end of match; striking candle on matchbox; blowing out candle and not match
3. Opening toothpaste, taking toothbrush from holder, and placing toothpaste on toothbrush.	Removing cap from toothpaste and placing cap on toothbrush; putting toothpaste in a tootbrush holder; placing toothbrush back in holder with tootpaste on it

In each of these tasks, the patient can usually perform each part of the series adequately (e.g., striking the match or brushing the teeth) but cannot coordinate the individual movements that are necessary to complete the sequence.

Clinical Implications

Ideational apraxia is a complex disability that is usually seen in patients with bilateral brain disease. Any diffuse cortical disease, especially those diseases that affect the parietal lobes, may result in an ideational apraxia. Although the patient fails on a specific task (e.g., lighting a candle), it is obvious from watching the patient's performance that his or her failure is the result of a number of cognitive deficits. Many patients have elements of ideomotor apraxia, and almost all have some degree of constructional impairment and spatial disorientation. Memory and auditory comprehension may also be diminished.

One interesting element in the performance of patients with ideational apraxia is their apparent inability to recognize the use of objects. This failure to recognize objects and their use has been called an object agnosia or a form of conceptual apraxia and may be illustrated by the patient who attempts to light a candle by striking it on the matchbox. The ability to do serial ordering is also impaired, and the complex multistep task becomes a confusing group of discrete parts with no logical, sequential relationship. The ambiguity and incongruity of the formal test situation also are confusing. The patient does not quite understand exactly what he or she is supposed to do when the doctor brings out a toothbrush and toothpaste and pushes it benignly toward the patient.

Neuropsychologically, ideational apraxia is the culmination of many significant cognitive deficits. Clinically, it results in the patient's inability to manipulate the environment effectively. The patient cannot cook a meal, make a bed, light a cigarette, use the channel changer on the TV, or do any of the dozens of everyday activities that we all take for granted. *Ideational apraxia is not usually seen in isolation but is generally associated with the widespread intellectual deterioration seen in patients with dementia, especially Alzheimer's disease.*

SUBCORTICAL COGNITIVE CHANGE

Considerable attention has been paid recently to the mental status changes occurring with disease that primarily affects the subcortical structures of the cerebral hemispheres (e.g., thalamus, putamen, globus pallidus, septal nucleus). *Diseases that primarily affect the subcortical structures include focal infarcts and trauma, Huntington's disease, progressive supranuclear palsy, and, more recently, acquired immunodeficiency syndrome (AIDS).* Mental status changes may be the defining illness in patients with AIDS; therefore, a specific battery of tests has been developed to diagnose this subcortical dementia.[45] *The main feature of subcortical dementia that differs from other dementias is psychomotor slowness.* Various tests of psychomotor speed can be used, but a quick and reliable test is to ask the patient to write the alphabet in uppercase letters. Normal individuals should be able to perform this test in under 21 seconds.[45]

RIGHT-LEFT DISORIENTATION

Right-left orientation is traditionally defined as the ability to distinguish right from left on oneself and in the environment (e.g., on the examiner's body). This ability is basically a capacity for spatial orientation.[9] The application of the verbal labels "right" and "left" to the respective sides of the body is frequently used to test right-left orientation,[32] but this is a linguistic task that does not necessarily test spatial sense. Right-left disorientation may be developmental in nature or may result from either focal or diffuse brain lesions. Although this disorder is interesting and may be combined with other deficits to produce Gerstmann's syndrome (discussed later in this chapter), it is of limited clinical utility when seen in isolation.

Evaluation

The following outline, which is in ascending order of difficulty, may be used to test for right-left disorientation.

TEST ITEMS
1. Identification on self
   A. Show me your right foot.
   B. Show me your left hand.
2. Crossed commands on self
   A. With your right hand touch your left shoulder.
   B. With your left hand touch your right ear.
3. Identification on examiner (with examiner facing patient)
   A. Point to my left knee.
   B. Point to my right elbow.
4. Crossed commands on examiner (with examiner facing patient)
   A. With your right hand point to my left eye.
   B. With your left hand point to my left foot.

Most normal persons will successfully accomplish all items without difficulty, although a significant percentage of the normal population (9% of males and over 17% of females) has demonstrable difficulty on right-left testing.[4,6]

Clinical Implications

If right-left disorientation is present, it is important to determine if the patient was ever capable of adequately performing such tasks. As previously mentioned, right-left disorientation may be developmental in nature and may also be associated with reduced general intellectual ability.

Aphasic patients may fail on right-left commands because of their primary language disorder. Anomia can cause confusion in the use of the labels "right" and "left." Deficits in auditory retention interfere with performance on complex commands.

Thus far, *clinical and neuropathologic case studies have failed to demonstrate an association between right-left disorientation and any circumscribed brain lesion.[24] If an acquired disorder of right-left orientation is present, the lesion is usually located in the parietotemporal-occipital region of the dominant hemisphere.[34]* In our clinical experience, right-left disorientation is infrequent in patients with lesions that are restricted to the nondominant hemisphere. This is also substantiated by Critchley's review.[9]

FINGER AGNOSIA

Finger agnosia is the inability to recognize, name, and point to individual fingers on oneself and on others.[25] This disorder may be most readily demonstrated in reference to the index, middle, and ring fingers.[8] Finger agnosia is similar to right-left orientation in that it may be developmental in nature or may result from either diffuse or focal brain disease. Its clinical utility for localization of cerebral lesions is relatively limited.

Evaluation

Evaluation of this function can be very extensive, but for practical purposes a brief screening should suffice. Patients must have adequate auditory comprehension and must know or be capable of learning the names of the fingers (thumb, index or pointing finger, middle finger, ring finger, and little finger).

TEST ITEMS

1. Nonverbal finger recognition

   Directions:
   With the patient's eyes closed, touch one finger. Have the patient open his or her eyes and then point to the same finger on the examiner's hand.

2. Identification of named fingers on examiner's hand

   Directions:
   The examiner's hand should be placed in various positions (e.g., palm down on the table facing the patient; hand held vertically in the air with the palm facing the patient; and hand held horizontally in the air with the palm facing the examiner). The examiner should say "Point to my middle finger," and so forth.

3. Verbal identification (naming) of fingers on self and examiner

   Directions:
   The patient's and examiner's hands should be placed in the various positions as described earlier. The examiner points to the patient's index finger and says, "What is the name of this finger?" and so forth.

Clinical Implications

Patients with finger agnosia usually have lesions of the dominant hemisphere.[37] Left-handed patients or those with strong family histories of left-handedness may exhibit finger agnosia with lesions of either hemisphere. Parietal-occipital lesions are the most likely to cause finger agnosia.[42] As with right-left testing, aphasia will adversely affect verbally mediated performance. For a more comprehensive review of this topic, see references 9 and 37.

GERSTMANN'S SYNDROME

Gerstmann's syndrome is a classic, albeit controversial, neurologic syndrome. It consists of four major components: finger agnosia, right-left disorientation, dysgraphia, and dyscalculia. Most patients with this disorder, however, demonstrate additional neuropsychologic deficits, principally constructional impairment or mild aphasia. The syndrome has localizing value; the demonstration of all four elements indicates damage to the dominant parietal lobe or to bilateral parietal lobes.[47,50,51] For further information about this syndrome, see references 6, 12, and 51.

VISUAL AGNOSIA

Visual agnosia is a rare, acquired neurologic syndrome in which the patient is unable to recognize objects or pictures of objects presented visually. Visual acuity is adequate, mentation clear, and aphasia absent.[52]

Two major categories of visual agnosia have been described in the literature. In the first type, actual visual perception of the object is distorted to the point that recognition is impossible. Such patients cannot name or tell the use of an object when it is shown to them but can readily name and demonstrate the use of the object when it is placed in their hands. Kinesthetic cues provide sufficient information for recognition. To evaluate for the presence of visual agnosia, ask the patient to identify verbally common objects presented visually. If the patient fails to recognize the object, allow manipulation of the object. If the patient then readily identifies the object, the defect is in the visual system. It has been postulated that such patients have damage to the visual association cortex bilaterally (areas 18 and 19). Recent studies using positron emission tomography (PET) scanning have verified the damage to the temporo-occipital cortex bilaterally.[31] This type of visual agnosia (**apperceptive visual agnosia**) has been reported in a patient with anoxic encephalopathy secondary to carbon dioxide poisoning[5] and in patients with Alzheimer's disease.

The second variety of visual agnosia is called **associative visual agnosia**. Patients with this type of agnosia have adequate visual perception but their visual cortex is disconnected from the language area or visual memory stores. Accordingly, they can recognize the object and demonstrate its use, but they cannot name it. When unable to name an object, such patients are also unable to describe its use.[49] The precise neuropsychologic defect for this disorder is still not clear. Whether it is a disconnection syndrome or a syndrome of subtle perceptual problems plus specific visual memory deficits remains to be elucidated. The evaluation for this disorder is similar to that for the first type of visual agnosia, except that adequate visual perception must be demonstrated. This can be done with a simple visual matching task. Lesions that cause an associative visual agnosia may be bilateral, involving the inferior temporal occipital junction and subjacent white matter,[2] or may be an infarct that destroys the left occipital lobe and the posterior corpus callosum.[38] This is the same lesion that causes alexia without agraphia, and, in fact, most patients with associative visual agnosia are also alexic. For further reading, see references 1, 2, 4, 10, and 38.

Two additional types of visual agnosia deserve mention but will not be fully discussed. **Prosopagnosia** is an unusual agnosia in which patients are unable to recognize familiar faces. In such cases, the agnosia is so profound that even members of the patient's immediate family are not recognized. The patient will recognize the person, however, on hearing his or her voice. The mechanism that results in prosopagnosia is probably a combination of a disturbance of fine visual discrimination and a failure of memory for the discrete category of human faces. The lesions that are responsible for this disorder are usually in the occipitotemporal areas bilaterally. One of the lesions is usually in the right inferior temporo-occipital region.[39] For further discussion, see references 7, 13, 16, 21, and 39.

Color agnosia is an inability to recognize colors secondary to an acquired cortical lesion. Two types of color agnosia have been described. A specific color-naming disturbance results from a disconnection of visual input from the language area. This anomia is associated with the syndrome of alexia with agraphia.[29] In this form, there is no damage to the primary language area and no other evidence of aphasia.

The second and more common disturbance of color recognition is actually a defect in color perception caused by bilateral inferior temporo-occipital lesions. These are the same lesions that cause prosopagnosia, and most patients with this type of color agnosia have concomitant prosopagnosia.[40] For further reading on this topic, refer to references 11 and 17.

ASTEREOGNOSIS

Stereognosis is the ability to discriminate the size and shape of objects and to identify them by touch alone. This is usually tested during the routine neurologic examination by asking the patient to identify several common objects placed in his or her hand (e.g., coin, key, paper clip, and so forth). The patient is tested with the eyes closed and is given one object at a time. The patient is allowed to manipulate the object freely. Each hand is tested individually.[9,33]

The task demands that the patient be able to integrate spatial features, weight, and texture in order to identify the object. If a patient has a defect in primary sensation in the hand, failure to identify the object cannot be attributed to astereognosis.

Classic astereognosis, or a failure of tactile recognition (tactile agnosia), usually indicates a lesion in the anterior portion of the parietal lobe opposite the astereognostic hand.[48] Cases have been reported in which a unilateral lesion, either right or left, produced a bilateral defect.[9] A rare form of left-hand unilateral astereognosis has been reported in patients with a lesion in the anterior corpus callosum.[30]

GEOGRAPHIC DISORIENTATION

Geographic orientation is a complex ability that includes the patient's capacity to find his or her way in familiar environments, to localize places on maps or floor plans, and to find his or her way in new environments. A significant geographic disorientation will interfere with the patient's ability to live a normal life. Such patients are unable to travel alone outside of their home and may even become disoriented within their own houses.

Evaluation

History Obtained from Family

In evaluating geographic orientation, it is important to obtain historical information regarding the patient's ability to operate in familiar and unfamiliar environments outside of the formal testing situation. Such information is best obtained from family members rather than from the patient.

1. Does the patient become lost at work, in the neighborhood, or at home?
2. Has the patient become lost traveling to a less-frequented location (e.g., the inability to locate a restaurant not visited in a year)?
3. Does the patient have great difficulty orienting to new environments?

Localizing Places on a Map

Map localization is an abstract task that can quickly detect disturbances in geographic orientation. It is also useful when adequate historical information is unobtainable, and it is particularly useful in bringing out subtle defects in unilateral attention.[8]

DIRECTIONS: Have the patient draw a map of the United States. If he or she is unable to produce a recognizable representation, the doctor should draw one or provide a suitable outline. Ask the patient to locate the following cities on the map outline:

Denver
New York
San Francisco
New Orleans
Chicago

SCORING: In reviewing the patient's performance, the following factors should be considered: (1) Are coastal cities located on the coast? (2) Are the cities in the appropriate states? (3) Are all cities in one half of the map (either east or west)? (4) Are attempts made to locate all cities?

Ability to Orient Self in Hospital Environment

Information concerning patients' ability to orient themselves in the hospital may be obtained from nurses' reports and by observing the patients' capacity to find their bed, ward, and bathroom. For example, we saw a patient with communicating hydrocephalus and mild dementia who, on concluding a fifth office revisit, walked confidently into the closet.

Clinical Implications

Geographic disorientation has been clinically associated with parietal lobe disease,[9] although good clinicoanatomic studies are few. Of the studies available, there is some suggestion that right hemisphere lesions most frequently cause geographic difficulty.[35] Other studies, however, have failed to support this finding of lateralization and report an approximately equal incidence of geographic disorientation in patients with right and left hemisphere lesions.[8]

A consistent finding of clinical usefulness is that *patients with unilateral lesions tend to localize cities on the map toward the side of their lesion* (e.g., patients with left parietal lesions tend to place cities toward the west coast on the map outline). This appears to be a result of neglect of the contralateral visual field.[8] *A more generalized geographic disorientation is a frequent finding in patients with diffuse cortical disease and may be an early sign of dementing illness.*

Geographic orientation is probably not a unitary cortical function but a combination of more basic cognitive processes including visual memory, right-left orientation, visual perception, and spatial neglect. Performance on formal tests of geographic orientation, such as locating cities on a map outline, is closely associated with both general intelligence and social exposure (education). *General lack of geographic knowledge is the most common cause of failure on the map test* and we were surprised to find that our normal subjects (on an average) correctly located only half of the five cities. Obviously, the effects of educational level (and quality), as well as social experience and exposure, are highly significant factors that must be considered when assessing geographic orientation.

One must not minimize the devastating effects that clinically significant geographic disorientation has on the patient's ability to function effectively. Such patients are typically unable to work, easily become lost in unfamiliar places, and eventually have difficulty with orientation in even familiar settings such as the neighborhood and home.

SUMMARY

The cortical functions of apraxia, right-left disorientation, visual and finger agnosia, astereognosis, and geographic disorientation are interesting and may be clinically relevant in localizing brain lesions.

REFERENCES

1. Albert, ML, Reches, A, and Silverberg, R: Associative visual agnosia without alexia. Neurology 25:322, 1975.
2. Alexander, MF and Albert, ML: The anatomical basis of visual agnosia. In Kertesz, A (ed): Localization in Neuropsychology. Academic Press, New York, 1983, pp 393–415.
3. Barbieri, C and DeRenzi, E: The executive and ideational components of apraxia. Cortex 24:535, 1988.
4. Bender, M and Feldman, M: The so-called "visual agnosias." Brain 95:173, 1972.
5. Benson, DF and Greenberg, J: Visual form agnosia. Arch Neurol 20:82, 1969.
6. Benton, A: The fiction of the Gerstmann syndrome. J Neurol Neurosurg Psychiatry 24:176, 1961.
7. Benton, A and Van Allen, M: Prosopagnosia and facial discrimination. J Neurol Sci 15:167, 1972.
8. Benton, A, Levin, H, and Van Allen, M: Geographic orientation in patients with unilateral cerebral disease. Neuropsychologia 12:183, 1974.
9. Critchley, M: The Parietal Lobes. Hafner, New York, 1966.
10. Critchley, M: The problem of visual agnosia. J Neurol Sci 1:274, 1964.
11. Critchley, M: Acquired anomalies of colour perception of central origin. Brain 88:711, 1965.
12. Critchley, M: The enigma of Gerstmann's syndrome. Brain 89:183, 1966.
13. Damasio, AR, Damasio, H, and Van Hoesen, GW: Prosopagnosia: Anatomic basis and behavioral mechanisms. Neurology 32:331, 1982.
14. DeAjuriaguerra, J, Hécaen, H, and Angelerques, R: Les apraxies: Variétés cliniques et lateralisation lésionnelle. Rev Neurol 102:566, 1960.
15. Denny-Brown, D: The nature of apraxia. J Nerv Ment Dis 126:9, 1958.
16. DeRenzi, E: Prosopagnosia. In Feinberg, TE and Farah, MN: Behavioral Neurology and Neuropsychology. McGraw-Hill, New York, 1997, pp 245–255.
17. DeRenzi, E, et al: Impairment in associating colour to form, concomitant with aphasia. Brain 95:293, 1972.
18. DeRenzi, E and Lucchelli, F: Ideational apraxia. Brain 111:1173, 1988.
19. DeRenzi, E, Motti, F, and Nichelli, P: Imitating gestures: A quantitative approach to ideomotor apraxia. Arch Neurol 37:6, 1980.
20. DeRenzi, E, Pieczuro, A, and Vignolo, L: Ideational apraxia: A quantitative study. Neuropsychologia 6:41, 1968.
21. DeRenzi, E and Spinnler, H: Facial recognition in brain damaged patients. Neurology 16:145, 1966.
22. Dewey, D: What is developmental dyspraxia? Brain Cogn 29:254–274,1995.
23. Foundas, AL, et al: Ecological implications of limb apraxia: Evidence from mealtime behaviors. Journal of the International Neurophysiological Society 1:62–66, 1995.
24. Frederiks, J: Disorders of the body schema. In Vinken, P and Bruyn, G (eds): Handbook of Clinical Neurology, Vol 4, Disorders of Speech, Perception and Symbolic Behavior. American Elsevier, New York, 1969, pp 207–240.
25. Gerstmann, J: Some notes on the Gerstmann-syndrome. Neurology 7:866, 1957.
26. Geschwind, N: Sympathetic dyspraxia. Trans Am Neurol Assoc 88:219, 1963.
27. Geschwind, N: Disconnection syndromes in animals and man, Part II. Brain 88:585, 1965.
28. Geschwind, N: The apraxias: Neural mechanisms of disorders of learned movement. Am Sci 63:188, 1975.
29. Geschwind, N and Fusillo, M: Color-naming defects in association with alexia. Arch Neurol 15:137, 1966.

30. Geschwind, N and Kaplan, E: A human cerebral deconnection syndrome. Neurology 12:675, 1962.
31. Grossman, M, Galetta, S, Ding X-S, et al: Clinical and positron emission tomography studies of visual apperceptive agnosia. Neuropsych Neuropsychol Behav Neurol 9:70–77, 1996.
32. Goodglass, H and Kaplan, E: The Assessment of Aphasia and Related Disorders, ed 2. Lea & Febiger, Philadelphia, 1983.
33. Hécaen, H and Albert, ML: Human Neuropsychology. John Wiley & Sons, 1978, pp 297–303.
34. Hécaen, H and DeAjuriaguerra, J: Méconnaissances et Hallucinations Corporelles. Masson et Cie., Paris, 1952.
35. Hécaen, H and Angelerques, R: La Cécite Psychique. Masson et Cie., Paris, 1963.
36. Heilman, KM, and Rothi, LJG. Apraxia. In Heilman, KM and Valenstein, E (eds). Clinical Neuropsychology, ed 3. Oxford University Press, New York, 1993, pp 141–163.
37. Kinsbourne, M and Warrington, E: A study of finger agnosia. Brain 85:47, 1962.
38. Lhermitte, F and Beauvois, M: A visual-speech disconnection syndrome. Brain 96:695, 1973.
39. Meadows, J: The anatomical basis of prosopagnosia. J Neurol Neurosurg Psychiatry 37:489, 1974.
40. Meadows, J: Disturbed perception of colours associated with localized cerebral lesions. Brain 97:615, 1974.
41. Nadeau, SE, Roeltgen, DP, Sevush, S, et al: Apraxia due to a pathologically documented thalamic infarction. Neurology 44:2133–2137, 1994.
42. Nielsen, J: Gerstmann syndrome: Finger agnosia, agraphia, confusion of right and left, and acalculia. Arch Neurol Psychiatry 39:536, 1983.
43. Ochipa, C, Rothi, LJG, Heilman, KM: Conceptual apraxia in Alzheimer's disease. Brain 115:1061–1071, 1992.
44. Poeck, K, Lehmkuhl, G, and Willmes, K: Axial movements in ideomotor apraxia. J Neurol Neurosurg Psychiatry 45:1125, 1982.
45. Power, C, Selnes, OA, Grim, JA. HIV dementia scale: A rapid screening test. J AIDS Hum Retrovirus 8:273–278, 1995.
46. Rapcsak, SZ, Ochipa, C, Beeson, PM, et al: Praxis and the right hemisphere. Brain Cogn 23:181-202, 1993.
47. Roeltgen, DP, Sevush, S, and Heilman, KM: Pure Gerstmann's syndrome from a focal lesion. Arch Neurol 40:46, 1983.
48. Roland, PE: Focal increase of cerebral blood flow during stereognostic testing in man. Arch Neurol 33:543, 1976.
49. Rubens, A and Benson, DF: Associative visual agnosia. Arch Neurol 24:305, 1971.
50. Strub, RL and Geschwind, N: Gerstmann syndrome without aphasia. Cortex 10:378, 1974.
51. Strub, RL and Geschwind, N: Localization in Gerstmann syndrome. In Kertesz, A (ed): Localization in Neuropsychology. Academic Press, New York, 1983, pp 295–321.
52. Warrington, EK: Agnosia: The impairment of object recognition. In Frederiks, JAM (ed): Handbook of Clinical Neurology, Vol 1(45), Clinical Neuropsychology. Elsevier Science, Amsterdam, 1985, pp 333–349.
53. Watson, RT, et al: Apraxia and the supplementary area. Arch Neurol 43:787, 1986.
54. Watson, RT and Heilman, KM: Callosal apraxia. Brain 106:391, 1983.
55. Wolf, SM: Difficulties in right-left discrimination in a normal population. Arch Neurol 29:128, 1973.

CHAPTER 10

SUMMARY OF EXAMINATION

Throughout this book, we have emphasized the importance of performing a systematic and complete mental status examination. Although it is not always necessary to evaluate exhaustively every aspect of mental functioning, *certain critical functions should be assessed in every patient.* These include:

- Level of consciousness
- Physical appearance and emotional status
- Attention
- Expressive and receptive language
- Memory
- Constructional ability
- Abstract reasoning

Items that are adequate for evaluating these areas are shown with an asterisk in the composite mental status examination shown in Appendix 2.

The experienced clinician can tailor the mental status examination to the individual patient's clinical problem and, with practice, can complete an adequate screening examination in 15 to 30 minutes. In patients with a vague history of behavioral complaints, or when emotional features predominate, a more extensive examination may be required.

The systematic mental status examination usually allows the clinician to differentiate patients with organic brain disease from both normal persons and those with functional disorders. In many cases, it is also possible to specify the type, locus, and degree of disease. For example, knowledge of specific patterns of aphasia often permits the examiner to localize a lesion within the dominant hemisphere. In other cases, the pattern of performance is suggestive of a specific disease entity (e.g., Alzheimer's disease).

In the Clinical Implications sections of each chapter in this book, we have attempted to describe many neurobehavioral syndromes as they relate to specific areas of cognitive deficit. Examples of these are the acute confusional states (Chapter 2), aphasias and related language disorders (Chapter 5), amnesias (Chapter 6), and the frontal lobe syndrome (Chapter 2) These sections of the text are not intended to be a comprehensive review of neurobehavior or an extensive discussion of any one syndrome, but should illustrate the bridge between the data and the diagnosis. See references 1, 3, and 8 for complete discussions of these topics.

In general, the more clinical data the examiner obtains regarding the patient's level of functioning in a variety of areas, the more accurate the final diagnosis will be. An examination that includes all of the items discussed in this book (outlined in Appendix 2) can usually be completed in an hour or less. Although all of the data are valuable, the busy clinician may not be able to spend this much time on all routine consultations. In most clinical settings, the initial goal is to make a tentative diagnosis and plan an appropriate diagnostic evaluation, so the examination will be tailored to fit the clinical situation. Following are discussions of several specific clinical neurobehavioral syndromes. Because of the magnitude of the problem of dementia, a disproportionate amount of space is devoted to the use of the mental status examination in diagnosing that condition.

ALZHEIMER'S DISEASE

One of the most common organic brain disorders is dementia,[4] and Alzheimer's disease (senile dementia Alzheimer type [SDAT]) is the most prevalent and well-known cause.[4,5,9] Although a cure is not yet available, it is important to recognize the early features of this syndrome because early diagnosis can prevent serious social and vocational embarrassment to both patient and family. *The early features of this disease are apathy, vague subjective complaints, decreased verbal fluency, memory difficulties, constructional impairment, dyscalculia (calculation problems), and problems with abstract reasoning.* As the disease progresses, anomia, apraxia, agnosia, geographic disorientation, and significant deficits in judgment typically appear, while the defects seen in the early stages worsen. In the deteriorated stage, all deficits are accentuated; behavior is regressed; language, memory, and thought processes are severely disturbed; and the patient requires total care. The diagnosis of Alzheimer's disease in the advanced stages is usually made without difficulty, but mild significant dementia can go unrecognized or misinterpreted by family members and health professionals alike.

The mental status examination for a patient with suspected dementia can be shortened but should include the following essential components:

1. **Level of consciousness:** Patients with simple atrophic dementia (Alzheimer's and senile Alzheimer's disease) are fully alert unless they

have a secondary decrease in the level of consciousness from medication, medical illness, or a focal brain lesion with increased intracranial pressure.

2. **Behavior observations:** These are important, but as they are made throughout the history and examination, they rarely prolong examination time.

3. **Language:** Spontaneous speech and comprehension can be roughly assessed during history taking, but verbal fluency, repetition, and naming should be specifically tested. Although naming and word-finding errors are often present in patients with dementia, repetition is usually intact unless the disease is advanced or there is an associated left hemisphere lesion with aphasia.

4. **Memory:** This is a critical term. Orientation should be tested first. If the patient fails, particularly if the failure is significant, this strongly suggests a new-learning or recent-memory deficit. Next, tell the patient the correct date and location and ask him or her to remember it. Then ask about recent news items for a few minutes, and then ask the orientation questions again. If there is a second failure, in our experience the patient has a significant memory problem, and additional testing will only support this initial impression and will not provide additional substantive data. If the patient is oriented or quickly learns his or her orientation, carry out the full memory section of the examination.

5. **Drawings:** These take only a few minutes to perform and are an invaluable aid in diagnosing brain disease, especially dementia.

6. **Abstract functions**
   1. **Calculations:** These are very useful when evaluating patients with dementia; several examples should be included.
   2. **Proverbs and similarities:** These are also useful, and several of each should be asked. The patient with dementia tends to provide very concrete answers.

After many years of use and the statistical analysis of hundreds of cases of Alzheimer's disease, the shortened form of the mental status examination shown in Table 10–1 was developed. The items were selected on the basis of sensitivity in diagnosing dementia. These items, although not specific to Alzheimer's disease, are highly likely to be abnormal in that population (i.e., highly sensitive). The total score for this test is 100 points (Table 10–2). Because of the potential for false-positive results in elderly persons (i.e., diagnosing dementia in nondemented individuals), a total score in the 50 to 60 range in an 85-year-old must be interpreted cautiously (Table 10–3).

TABLE 10-1. Mental Status Examination for Dementia

PATIENT INFORMATION

NAME: DATE:

HOSPITAL OR FILE NUMBER:

AGE: SEX: DIAGNOSIS:

1. VERBAL FLUENCY

   Animals per 60 seconds   Total animals: _____

2. COMPREHENSION   Check if correct:

   a. Point to the ceiling.   _____

   b. Point to your nose and window.   _____

   c. Point to your foot, door, and ceiling.   _____

   d. Point to window, leg, door, and thumb.   _____

3. NAMING AND WORD FINDING

   Parts of objects: Watch stem (winder)   _____

                              Coat lapel   _____

                              Watch crystal   _____

                              Sole of shoe   _____

                              Buckle of belt   _____

4. ORIENTATION

   a. Date   _____

   b. Month   _____

   c. Year   _____

   d. Day of week   _____

5. NEW LEARNING ABILITY

   Four unrelated words: 5 min   10 min

   a. Brown (Fun) (Grape)   _____   _____

   b. Honesty (Loyalty) (Happiness)   _____   _____

   c. Tulip (Carrot) (Stocking)   _____   _____

   d. Eyedropper (Ankle) (Toothbrush)   _____   _____

6. VERBAL STORY FOR IMMEDIATE RECALL

   It was July / and the Rogers / had packed up / their four children / in the station wagon / and were off / on vacation.

   They were taking / their yearly trip / to the beach / at Gulf Shores.

   This year / they were making / a special / one-day stop / at The Aquarium / in New Orleans.

   After a long day's drive / they arrived / at the motel / only to discover / that in their excitement / they had left / the twins / and their suitcases / in the front yard.

   Number of correct memories: _____

149

TABLE 10-1.	**Mental Status Examination for Dementia** *(Continued)*

7. VISUAL MEMORY (HIDDEN OBJECTS)

Object   Found

  a. Coin   _____
  b. Pen   _____
  c. Comb   _____
  d. Key   _____
  e. Fork   _____

8. PAIRED ASSOCIATE LEARNING

	1		2
a.	Weather—Box	a.	House—Income
b.	High—Low	b.	Weather—Box
c.	House—Income	c.	Book—Page
d.	Book—Page	d.	High—Low

	1		2
a.	House _____	a.	High _____
b.	High _____	a.	House _____
c.	Weather _____	c.	Book _____
d.	Book _____	d.	Weather _____

9. CONSTRUCTIONAL ABILITY

Score _____

Daisy in flower pot   Score _____

House in perspective   Score _____

TABLE 10-1.	**Mental Status Examination for Dementia** **(*Continued*)**

10. WRITTEN COMPLEX
    CALCULATIONS

    a. Addition

$$108 \atop {+\ 79}$$

    b. Subtraction

$$605 \atop {-\ 86}$$

    c. Multiplication

$$108 \atop {\times\ 36}$$

    d. Division $43\overline{)559}$ Number correct _____

11. PROVERB INTERPRETATION

    a. Don't cry over spilled milk.   Score

    b. Rome wasn't built in a day.

    c. A drowning man will clutch at a straw.

    d. A golden hammer can break down an iron door.

    e. The hot coal burns, the cold one blackens.

12. SIMILARITIES

    a. Turnip .... Cauliflower   _____

    b. Car .... Airplane   _____

    c. Desk .... Bookcase   _____

    d. Poem .... Novel   _____

    e. Horse .... Apple

TABLE 10-2. **Mental Status Scoresheet**

PATIENT:				Score
Verbal fluency—animal names (1 point/2 animals)			Maximum: 10 points	_____
Verbal comprehension (pointing)			4 points	_____
Naming—parts of objects			5 points	_____
Memory				
Orientation:	Date	2 points	6 points	_____
	Day	2 points		
	Month	1 point		
	Year	1 point		
Unrelated words (2 points each) 5 min _____ 10 min _____			16 points	_____
Story (1 point = 1 remembered item [13 maximum])			13 points	_____
Hidden objects (1 point each)			5 points	_____
Paired associate learning			8 points	_____
Drawings Pipe, daisy, house			9 points	_____
Calculations (written)			4 points	_____
Proverbs			10 points	_____
Similarities			10 points	_____
			Maximum: 100 points	_____

TABLE 10-3. **Total Scores on Mental Status Examination for Dementia**

Normal Individuals

Age Group	Mean Score (standard deviation)
40–49	80.9 (9.7)
50–59	82.3 (8.6)
60–69	75.5 (10.5)
70–79	66.9 (9.1)
80–89	67.9 (11.0)

Patients with Alzheimer's Disease

Stage	Mean Score (standard deviation)
I	57.2 (9.1)
II	37.0 (7.8)
III	13.4 (8.1)

ACUTE CONFUSIONAL STATE

A history of a rapid decrease in mental status (hours to a few days) does not usually suggest a primary dementia but more likely a delirium (acute confusional state). As discussed in Chapter 2, this condition is usually easily recognized by its typical behavioral features and represents a specific diagnostic entity. Extensive mental status testing usually yields abnormal results but rarely adds additional useful diagnostic information.

LESIONS OF THE DOMINANT HEMISPHERE

Patients with lesions of the dominant hemisphere frequently show abnormalities of language functions. In the right-handed patient, evidence of aphasia, alexia, or agraphia almost always indicates left hemisphere disease. Gerstmann's syndrome, constructional impairment, verbal memory difficulties, ideomotor apraxia, dyscalculia, and impairment of verbal reasoning are all findings that can be seen with left hemisphere lesions. Denial and neglect are not commonly seen in these patients. Even left-handed patients frequently show the aforementioned findings with left hemisphere disease, although there is a higher frequency of bilateral representation of these functions in these patients.

LESIONS OF THE NONDOMINANT HEMISPHERE

Although most patients with lesions of the nondominant hemisphere do not show evidence of language disorders, they do have a more dramatic constructional impairment than do patients with dominant-hemisphere lesions. In such patients, denial and neglect are more common and severe in degree, malalignment is seen in writing and calculations, and deficits are present in nonverbal memory.

AIDS DEMENTIA

In AIDS dementia, the cognitive areas most commonly impaired are attention, psychomotor speed, and recent memory, but it is always prudent to assess constructional facility, proverb interpretation, and reading ability.

RECORDING, SUMMARIZING, AND INTERPRETING DATA

As with any medical examination, *it is very important to record both what was specifically tested and the patient's responses to each item.* A form similar to the composite in Appendix 2 should be used as an aid in recording these data. At the completion of the examination, the clinician should synthesize the data and then summarize and emphasize the key areas of impairment. This summary allows an identification of deficit patterns and the efficient communication of essential findings.

The clinician must summarize and organize the data in such a way that he or she can arrive at the following four clinical implications:

1. **Describe the major areas of impairment:** Indicate those areas of mental status functioning that are deficient compared with the level expected in the patient, based on his or her education and premorbid function (e.g., verbal memory, abstraction, or construction ability). This is the initial step in organizing the data so that they can be interpreted neurobehaviorally.

2. **Make a tentative neurobehavioral diagnosis:** Having indicated the major areas of impairment, the clinician can now analyze the pattern of deficits and make a specific neurobehavioral diagnosis: delirium, dementia, organic amnesic state, aphasia, nondominant-hemisphere syndrome, and so forth. The interpretation of the mental status findings is difficult and, as in all fields of medicine, requires clinical experience with patients who have organic brain syndromes (neurobehavioral disorders), as well as additional reading in this area.

3. **Arrive at a tentative localization of the lesion:** This step is of both practical and academic importance. In a practical sense, findings that suggest a single focal lesion (e.g., fluent aphasia without other deficits, suggesting a left temporal or temporoparietal lesion) require a far different neurodiagnostic evaluation than does the identification of a global cognitive disorder such as an acute confusional state or dementia. Academically it is of great interest to attempt to correlate clinical findings with what is known about brain function.

4. **Make a tentative clinical diagnosis:** This is the final step in the diagnostic process. It requires the clinician to correlate historical and examination data with medical knowledge to make a specific medical diagnosis. For example, a patient with a slowly developing cognitive deterioration, whose mental status examination shows multiple areas of impairment suggesting bilateral brain disease (dementia), yet who has normal results on a standard neurologic examination, most likely has Alzheimer's disease. Similarly, an elderly patient with the acute onset of aphasia with fluent paraphasic speech with impaired comprehension (Wernicke's aphasia) probably has had an occlusion of a posterior branch of the left middle cerebral artery.

This entire summary process requires careful thought and considerable clinical knowledge. When the examiner becomes proficient with the examination and familiar with the organic syndromes, this complex process of data analysis and diagnosis becomes easier.

The final steps in any patient evaluation include communicating test findings to the patient, the patient's family, and the referring physician; referring the patient for further evaluation when necessary; arranging for appropriate neurodiagnostic evaluation; and planning subsequent patient management.

SUMMARY

As stated in our introduction, we have intended to help the clinician to understand many of the cognitive functions that can be easily tested at the bedside. We have tried to give enough information concerning these functions and their disturbance in brain disease to allow the examiner to test the patient and to delineate the deficits. Understanding these deficits and how to test for them, and recognizing the common pattern in disease, often permits the examiner to make a specific diagnosis.

After reading this book, the neurologist, psychiatrist, psychologist, or other health care provider should be able to conduct a comprehensive examination of the patient with brain disease and use the data for diagnosis. Although this mental status examination is qualitative, it can be quantitative if the examiner so desires. Some screening tests (the Mini-Mental State Examination[1] being the most widely used) give the examiner a single score, which is used to identify the presence and degree of organic disease. This quantitative method, in contrast to the comprehensive qualitative examination, can provide only a gross estimate of the patient's global cognitive functioning and is restricted in its contents, scope, and sensitivity. A plethora of screening tests to identify dementia exists, from the 7 Minute Screen[7] to the test in which the patient must rearrange alphabetically the letters in the word "world."[6] All such tests assess cognitive level and can be useful for screening. This book is designed as an educational tool to help the examiner to understand the richness of cognitive functioning and its assessment. Selection of any number of individual items to test such as orientation, verbal fluency, and recall of five hidden objects can serve as an excellent screening test, but the information gained from these short tests is limited and should not be relied on in isolation.

REFERENCES

1. Feinberg, TE and Farah, MJ: Behavioral Neurology and Neuropsychology. McGraw-Hill, New York, 1997.
2. Folstein, MF, Folstein, SE, and McHugh, PR: "Mini-Mental State": A practical method for grading the cognitive state of patients for the clinician. J Psychiatr Res 12:189, 1975.
3. Heilman, KM and Valenstein, E: Clinical Neuropsychology, ed 3. Oxford University Press, New York, 1993.
4. Katzman, R: The prevalence and malignancy of Alzheimer's disease. Arch Neurol 33:217, 1976.

5. Katzman, R and Karasu, T: Differential diagnosis of dementia. In Fields, W (ed): Neurological and Sensory Disorders in the Elderly. Stratton Intercontinental Medical Books, New York, 1975, pp 103–134.
6. Leopold, NA and Borson, AJ: An alphabetical 'WORLD': A new version of an old test. Neurology 49:1521–1524, 1997.
7. Solomon, PR, et al: A 7 minute neurocognitive screening battery highly sensitive to Alzheimer's disease. Arch Neurol 55:349–355, 1998.
8. Strub, RL and Black, FW: Neurobehavioral Disorders: A Clinical Approach. FA Davis, Philadelphia, 1988.
9. Whitehouse, PJ (ed): Dementia. FA Davis, Philadelphia, 1992.

CHAPTER

11

FURTHER EVALUATIONS

In a number of patients, completion of the mental status examination prompts the need for one or more additional specialized evaluations or consultations. This section briefly discusses the contributions of the neuropsychologist, speech pathologist, psychiatrist, and social worker to the evaluation and management of the patient with organic brain damage or disease. It is beyond the scope of this book to offer more than a basic introduction to each specialty, with suggested readings for each area.

NEUROPSYCHOLOGY

Clinical neuropsychologists are trained at the doctoral level, with a 1-year clinical internship, a postdoctoral fellowship, or both, during which formal training is obtained in the evaluation and behavioral treatment of patients with organic brain disease. Reference 1 gives more detailed information regarding recommended training for neuropsychologists. Clinical neuropsychologists are primarily concerned with the identification, description, and quantification of changes in behavior (cognitive, motor, and emotional) that are associated with brain dysfunction. Their primary area of expertise is the investigation of the relationships between human behavior (whether a specific response on a formal test or in day-to-day functioning) and brain function and dysfunction. Accordingly, the neuropsychologist can aid in a variety of important clinical problems, including differential diagnosis, lateralization and localization of lesions, establishment of baselines of behavior and cognitive performance from which improvement or deterioration can be gauged, determination of competence in the aged or demented, and development of remedial methods for the rehabilitation of the individual brain-damaged patient.[7-9,17]

The neuropsychological evaluation is a comprehensive, objective assessment of a wide range of cognitive, adaptive, and emotional behaviors that reflect the adequacy (or inadequacy) of higher brain functions. In essence, the neuropsychological evaluation is a greatly expanded and objectified mental status examination. The mental status examination is designed to screen a variety of critical areas briefly, whereas the neuropsychological evaluation assesses a wider range of performance in considerably more depth. It differs from the mental status examination in that it generally uses tests and evaluation procedures that have been standardized with samples of either normal people or brain-damaged patients. Because of the use of standardized tests, the individual patient's performance can be compared to that of normative groups, and the adequacy of a patient's performance can be compared across a variety of neurobehavioral areas. The objective and highly quantified nature of most neuropsychological tests aids in the detection of subtle changes in performance over time (e.g., a slowly deteriorating dementia or the improvement in specific cognitive functions after epilepsy neurosurgery). Because of the wide range of behaviors assessed and the depth of the evaluation, the neuropsychological evaluation frequently can detect subtle deficits not apparent on the mental status examination.

Referral

Appropriate referrals for neuropsychological evaluation include patients in whom brain damage is suspected but not unequivocally verified, as well as those for whom the physician requires further information regarding diagnosis, description of the effects of a well-verified lesion on behavior, or prognosis and rehabilitation. As with any consultation, the questions that should be answered (e.g., "Is this patient demented or depressed?" or "Will the effects of this head injury interfere with the patient's ability to do his or her job?") should be stated as clearly as possible.

Cognitive and behavioral disturbances may occur in the absence of any clear-cut physical signs of cerebral disease on a standard clinical neurologic examination; this is particularly true in cases of early-stage progressive neurologic disease or mild closed-head injury. In cases of early dementia, the neuropsychological evaluation can often contribute to an appropriate diagnosis, in combination with other neurodiagnostic procedures. The dilemma of differentiating between dementia and depression is usually readily resolved by the data obtained from the neuropsychological assessment. In other cases, the neuropsychological evaluation can provide data suggestive of brain dysfunction, which then serve as a basis for completing a more extensive and specific neurodiagnostic workup.

The neuropsychological evaluation can also determine the relative impact of the organic and functional components in patients with mixed neurologic and psychiatric complaints, which occurs frequently in geriatric medicine.

Any patient with a documented brain lesion in whom rehabilitation is planned should receive a complete neuropsychological assessment as part of the initial comprehensive evaluation. This assessment provides valuable information regarding the effect of the lesion on cognitive functioning, emotional status, behavior, and social adjustment. Objective data document both specific areas of impairment and residual abilities. This outline of strengths and weaknesses is essential in providing information for planning cognitive, vocational, and social rehabilitation.

Periodic reevaluations over time provide reliable, objective information regarding the speed and degree of recovery after brain injury or the effectiveness of specific drug treatment regimens. Similarly, repeat evaluations can assess deterioration in patients with progressive disease or rule out such progression in equivocal cases. Testing before and after neurosurgery helps to quantify the effects of surgery on the patient's neurobehavioral functioning.

In any case of trauma or suspected brain damage involving litigation or compensation, the objective data obtained from a neuropsychological evaluation are of great value in documenting and describing the presence, absence, and degree of disability. There is considerable legal precedent for the admission of testimony of psychologists as expert witnesses in such cases. Forensic neuropsychology is a rapidly emerging subspecialty, requiring additional training and experience, which has proven very helpful to clinicians and attorneys alike dealing with cases of traumatically acquired brain damage.[6,8,24]

Contributions of the Neuropsychological Evaluation

The following summarize the major clinical contributions of the neuropsychological evaluation.

Categorization

Categorization provides information regarding the presence or absence of brain dysfunction, significant emotional disturbance, or both. The differential diagnosis among a primary organic, primary functional, or mixed disorder is made. If significant components of both organic and functional features are present, the relative impact of each will be discussed.

Localization

Performance on the neuropsychological test battery can be analyzed to provide data to determine if the brain dysfunction is diffuse or focal. Further analysis provides data regarding the lateralization of the lesion to the right or left hemisphere and localization of the lesion within the anterior or posterior region of the hemisphere. With the advent of new neurodiagnostic procedures (magnetic resonance imaging, positron emission tomography, etc.) this traditional focus of the neuropsychological evaluation has become less important clinically, although it continues to be of theoretical and research interest.

Description

The neuropsychological evaluation can provide a comprehensive description of the patient's current level of functioning in a wide range of cognitive, adaptive, emotional, and behavioral areas. This is perhaps the best use of neuropsychological consultation in many cases. A comprehensive overview of the patient's deficits and residual abilities describes current functioning, explains present behavior, determines the relative effects of organic and functional factors, and provides a baseline of data from which to judge future change. Answers to the question of mental competence and social independence can also be provided.

Prognosis and Recommendations

Based on the nature of the neurologic disease and the pattern and degree of deficits seen during the neuropsychological evaluation, a determination of the probability and degree of expected recovery or deterioration can be made for many patients. Reevaluation is very helpful in making valid prognostic statements in case of either progression or recovery. Further evaluations, including psychiatry, speech pathology, occupational therapy, and social service, may be recommended, as may specific remedial methods or programs.

Components

A meaningful review of the components of the neuropsychological evaluation is beyond the scope of this book; see references 2, 4, 17, and 25 for additional information regarding the specific tests used in the neuropsychological evaluation and further details about the field of clinical neuropsychology.

The amount of literature pertaining to clinical neuropsychology has increased almost exponentially during the past 20 years. The amount of available material forces the interested reader to be highly selective in choosing books that are both current and clinically pertinent. A representative selection might include references 2, 4, 8, 9, 11, 14, and 17.

SPEECH PATHOLOGY

Patients with significant difficulty in communicating, as a result of neurologic disease or injury (e.g., patients with aphasia, apraxia of speech, or dysarthria), should be evaluated by a speech pathologist. Not all such patients are treatment candidates, but, through thorough language evaluation, the speech pathologist can determine appropriate candidates for speech and language therapy and provide other services to patients who are not selected for treatment. The speech pathologist is an important member of any comprehensive rehabilitation team, particularly when a facility sees a large number of stroke and trauma patients.

Evaluation by the speech pathologist provides a description of the patient's communicative abilities and deficits, the possible benefits of therapeutic intervention, and a plan for family counseling to facilitate the development of alternative methods of communicating with the patient.

Referral

The major reasons for referring patients to a speech pathologist include:

- The mental status examination indicates a probable organic communication disorder that requires a more thorough evaluation.
- An obvious communication disorder exists that requires a screening evaluation to determine the appropriateness of speech therapy.
- A significant communication disorder is present that requires family counseling to inform the family members about the patient's problem and to assist in maximizing effective communication in the home.

For additional information regarding the important role of the speech pathologist in the evaluation and treatment of neurologic patients, see references 5, 10, 16, 20, and 23.

PSYCHIATRY

Many patients with organic brain disease have an associated emotional disorder that deserves psychiatric consultation. Patients appropriately referred for evaluation include those with the following:

- Psychiatric disorders that preceded their neurologic problem
- Neurologically based emotional problems (e.g., organic mood disorder)
- Emotional reactions to brain disease or trauma (e.g., adjustment disorder)
- Emotional factors complicating dementia
- Functional disorders that present as neurologic conditions (e.g., conversion disorder paralysis)[3]

Emotional factors are frequently significant in the rehabilitation and social reintegration of the patient with organic disease. A psychiatrist or psychologist should be consulted to aid in the management of any patient with an emotional problem severe enough to interfere with rehabilitative efforts or home adjustment.

Referral

Because of the relatively high incidence of both mental illness and brain disease, many patients have coexisting psychiatric and neurologic conditions (e.g., a brain tumor in a schizophrenic patient, a seizure patient with a manic-depressive disorder). For instance, we saw a 37-year-old woman with a long premorbid psychiatric history. The patient also suffered from alcoholism and over the years had sustained several significant traumatic head injuries. After alcohol withdrawal, she had several grand mal seizures and was admitted to the neurology ward. As her postictal confusion cleared, she demonstrated gross delusional and aggressive behavior. A complete history and medical evaluation indicated that the patient had an acute neurologic condition superimposed on a preexisting schizophrenia. Because of the underlying psychosis, a psychiatrist was consulted for treatment and long-term management.

It is not uncommon for previously emotionally stable individuals to develop a significant emotional reaction to an acute-onset neurobehavioral disorder such as aphasia. Depressive reactions, anxiety, paranoia, and aggressiveness may develop in response to brain damage. Such emotional responses often significantly interfere with rehabilitation efforts and require appropriate evaluation and treatment.

Patients with dementia present a particular challenge because of their combined intellectual and emotional changes. These changes produce a variety of difficult management problems that are often best handled with the aid of a geriatric psychiatrist or neuropsychiatrist. In the early stage of dementia, patients may retain considerable insight; this capacity to realize the seriousness of their condition often results in profound depression. Other patients with dementia are unaware of their deteriorating intellectual ability; such patients often push themselves beyond their capability and thus develop reactive frustration and severe anxiety. Anxiety or depression can greatly exacerbate the mental and social disability experienced by the patient with dementia. The psychiatrist can provide great assistance through the use of psychotropic drugs, family counseling, and general patient management.

Patients with chronic organic mental syndromes such as significant dementia, severe traumatic encephalopathy, or Korsakoff's disease may become management problems and eventually require long-term placement in chronic-care facilities. Early referral to the psychiatrist or medical social worker can help the family and the primary care clinician with the administrative and legal details involved in such placement.

A final group of patients who may initially be seen by the neurologist, but who require referral to a mental health professional for treatment, are those with somatoform disorders (e.g., conversion disorders or pseudodementia). Such patients will present with symptoms that mimic neurologic disease (e.g., limb paralysis, loss of speech, or sensory loss) but demonstrate no organic etiology after thorough evaluation. The treatment for such functional disorders is most often psychotherapy in association with psychotropic medication.

Information regarding specific psychiatric interview, evaluation, and treatment techniques is readily available in all major texts.[13,28]

SOCIAL WORK

In dealing with neurologic patients and their families in either postacute hospital settings or long-term follow-up and rehabilitation, social workers are important resources for better patient management. The primary areas of social work input in such settings include:

- Gathering and evaluating premorbid, psychosocial, and family information, crucial to understanding the patient and the effect of the neurologic illness or trauma on the patient's ability to function
- Participating in patient management and family education and support processes during the early recovery stage
- Serving as the primary data collator, resource investigator, and coordinator of the referral and placement process when considering a rehabilitation or long-term care facility

Although not all patients and families need all aspects of the social worker's total role, virtually all can benefit from some degree of involvement. See Johnson and McCown[12] for an overview of the role of family therapy in dealing with neurologic patients and their families, and Thyer and Wodarski[26] for a more comprehensive introduction to the various roles of the social worker in managing patients with neurobehavioral disorders.

COGNITIVE REHABILITATION

In recent decades, the fields of cognitive retraining and neurorehabilitation have become prominent, albeit somewhat controversial, forces in the treatment of brain-injured patients. Providing specific therapies (e.g., physical, speech-language, psychologic) to promote maximal recovery of particular neurobehavioral deficits after traumatic brain injury or an acute neurologic event (e.g., stroke) is not new, but only in the last 20 years or so have comprehensive rehabilitation programs become readily available to such patients. Discussion of the theoretical framework underlying specific cognitive retraining orientations and the nature of comprehensive programs, as well as the practical logistics, advantages, and problems of cognitive rehabilitation programs, is beyond the scope of this book. However, the clinician dealing with patients suffering from static neurologic disorders and traumatically induced neurobehavioral deficits should become acquainted with this rapidly evolving area as a potential patient-treatment resource. Decisions regarding whom to refer, when to refer, and particularly where to refer are difficult and should be approached with considerable understanding of the developments in this field and an awareness of the positive and negative aspects of particular programs. We suggest references 15, 19, 21, 22, and 27 for good introductions to and critical reviews of this important field.

SUMMARY

The management of patients with organic brain disease is a multidisciplinary effort. Physicians and other health professionals are strongly encouraged to acquaint themselves with the expertise and clinical services offered by their colleagues in related specialized fields, who can help in understanding patients better and providing them with more comprehensive and effective evaluation and treatment.

REFERENCES

1. Adams, KM and Rourke, BP (eds): The TCN Guide to Professional Practice in Clinical Neuropsychology. Swets and Zeitlinger, Berwyn, PA, 1992.
2. Adams, RL, et al (eds): Neuropsychology for Clinical Practice. American Psychology Association, Washington, DC, 1997.
3. American Psychiatric Association: Diagnostic and Statistical Manual of Mental Disorders, ed 4 (DSM-IV). American Psychiatric Press, Washington, DC, 1994.
4. Anderson, RM: Practitioner's Guide to Clinical Neuropsychology. Plenum Press, New York, 1994.
5. Benson, DF and Ardila, A: Aphasia: A Clinical Perspective. Oxford University Press, New York, 1996.
6. Doerr, HO and Carlin, AS: Forensic Neuropsychology. Guilford Press, New York, 1991.
7. Feinberg, TE and Farah, MJ (eds): Behavioral Neurology and Neuropsychology. McGraw-Hill, New York, 1996.
8. Filskov, SB and Boll, TJ (eds): Handbook of Clinical Neuropsychology. Wiley-Interscience, New York, 1981.
9. Filskov, SB and Boll, TJ (eds): Handbook of Clinical Neuropsychology, Vol II. Wiley-Interscience, New York, 1986.
10. Goodglass, H and Kaplan, E: The Assessment of Aphasia and Related Disorders, ed 2. Lea & Febiger, Philadelphia, 1983.
11. Heilman, KM and Valenstein, E (eds): Clinical Neuropsychology, ed 3. Oxford University Press, New York, 1993.
12. Johnson, J and McCown, W: Family Therapy of Neurobehavioral Disorders: Integrating Neuropsychology and Family Therapy. Haworth Press, Binghamton, NY, 1997.
13. Kaplan, HI and Sadock, BJ: Comprehensive Textbook of Psychiatry, ed 6. Williams & Wilkins, Baltimore, 1995.
14. Kolb, B and Whishaw, IQ: Fundamentals of Human Neuropsychology, ed 4. WH Freeman, New York, 1995.
15. Kreutzer, JS and Wehman, P (eds): Cognitive Rehabilitation for Persons with Traumatic Brain Injury. Imaginart, Bisbee, AZ, 1996.
16. Lapoint, LL (ed): Aphasia and Related Neurogenic Language Disorders. Thieme Medical Publishers, New York, 1996.
17. Lezak, MD: Neuropsychologic Assessment, ed 3. Oxford University Press, New York, 1995.
18. McCaffrey, RJ, et al (eds): The Practice of Forensic Neuropsychology. Plenum Press, New York, 1997.
19. Meier, M, Benton, A, and Diller, L: Neuropsychologic Rehabilitation. Guilford Press, New York, 1987.
20. Plum, F (ed): Language, Communication, and the Brain. Raven Press, New York, 1988.
21. Prignatano, GP: Learning from our successes and failures: Reflections and comment on "Cognitive Rehabilitation: How it is and how it might be." Journal of the International Neuropsychologic Society 3:497, 1997.
22. Rosenthal, M, et al (eds): Rehabilitation of the Adult and Child with Traumatic Brain Injury, ed 2. FA Davis, Philadelphia, 1990.
23. Sarno, MT (ed): Acquired Aphasia, ed 2. Academic Press, New York, 1991.

24. Spordone, RJ: Neuropsychology for the Attorney. Paul Deutch Press, Orlando, 1991.

25. Spreen, O and Strauss, E: A Compendium of Neuropsychologist Tests, ed 2. Oxford University Press, New York, 1997.

26. Thyer, BA and Wodarski, JS (eds): Handbook of Empirical Social Work Practice. John Wiley and Sons, New York, 1998.

27. Wilson, BA: Cognitive rehabilitation: How it is and how it might be. Journal of the International Neuropsychologic Society 3:487, 1997.

28. Yudofsky, SC and Hales, RE (eds): Textbook of Neuropsychiatry. American Psychiatric Press, Washington, DC, 1997.

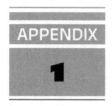

STANDARD NEUROPSYCHOLOGICAL ASSESSMENT METHODS

The primary purpose of this appendix is to introduce the physician and other specialists to psychological tests that are commonly encountered in neuropsychological reports and that have proved to be clinically useful in the assessment of patients with neurologic dysfunction. It is not intended as a comprehensive overview of neuropsychological evaluation procedures or as an in-depth evaluation of any individual test or technique. See references 11, 28, 39, or 44 for such detailed information.

FIXED BATTERY VERSUS FLEXIBLE ASSESSMENT APPROACHES

The two primary underlying philosophic approaches to neuropsychological assessment at this time are the fixed battery and flexible assessment methods. The fixed battery typically consists of a standard series of neuropsychological tests, each of which is administered to every patient regardless of the presenting complaint or specific findings obtained during the course of the assessment. This approach grew out of the American psychometric approach to psychological and neuropsychological evaluation. Most neuropsychologists augment the fixed battery with additional tests to more carefully evaluate a particular problem if it becomes apparent during the evaluation. The Halstead-Reitan Neuropsychologic Battery is the most representative of the fixed batteries, although few psychologists currently use this approach without the addition of various other measures.

The flexible approach most commonly uses a small core battery of tests to provide an overview of the patient's functioning and to suggest particular areas of neurobehavioral function that may require more definitive evaluation. Accordingly, it is a much more individualized approach, with the actual battery of tests to be administered varying from patient to patient, depending on the particular set of clinical questions raised. This "process" assessment approach is more akin to the single-sample method of Luria and to behavioral neurology than to the more traditional standard methods of clinical neuropsychology. The Wechsler Adult Intelligence Scale–Revised as a Neuropsychological Instrument (WAIS-RNI)[22] and Christensen's adaptation of Luria's techniques[6] are representative of this philosophic approach. In reality, the well-trained neuropsychologist typically uses elements of both underlying philosophies in the selection of particular tests for an individual battery, in the general approach to patient evaluation, and in the analysis of test results.

COMPREHENSIVE FIXED BATTERIES

Halstead-Reitan Battery

This battery, comprising a well-standardized series of tests of cognitive and adaptive ability, was originally introduced by Halstead,[15] revised and standardized by Reitan and associates, and statistically refined by Reitan and Wolfson,[35] Russell and colleagues,[37] and others.[18] The core tests included in this battery include: (1) the Category Test, (2) Tactual Performance Test, (3) Seashore Rhythm Test, (4) Speech-Sounds Perception Test, and (5) Finger-Oscillation (Finger-Tapping) Test. Age-graded norms for the basic Halstead-Reitan Battery and for many additional tests frequently used in conjunction with this battery are now available.[18] The primary limitations of the Halstead-Reitan Battery include its length, its limited emphasis on important neurobehavioral areas such as memory and language, and a lack of test results that can be readily translated to functionally relevant descriptive information useful to the patient, physician, and others involved in patient care. Its primary intent, which is to diagnose brain dysfunction and not to delineate and describe functional disabilities, appears somewhat dated in an era of magnetic resonance imaging (MRI) for anatomic visualization and positron emission tomography (PET) to assess physiologic functioning of the brain. However, as typically augmented by the addition of tests of general cognitive ability, language, and memory, this battery remains one of the best and most popular standardized methods of identifying patients with neurologic dysfunction. See references 21 and 35 for more detailed information on this assessment technique.

Luria-Nebraska Neuropsychological Battery

This battery,[11] which was an attempt to standardize and provide normative data on selected items adapted from the Christensen-Luria materials, has been the source of both considerable clinical popularity and major criticism in the neuropsychological literature since its inception. It represents a standardized fixed battery application of a basically flexible approach, and accordingly incorporates some of the best and most of the worst features of both methods. Although the battery is still available and is used by some clinicians, it is no longer well accepted nor in frequent clinical or forensic use.[27]

TESTS COMMONLY USED IN FIXED AND FLEXIBLE BATTERIES

Luria's Neuropsychological Investigation

Christensen[6] organized some of Luria's materials and techniques into a written format, with a manual of administration instructions, within a framework that corresponded to his conceptualization of brain function—behavior relationships. This has allowed the well-trained clinician to use and adapt Luria's experimental procedures for clinical patient examination. It is perhaps the foremost example of the flexible assessment approach. The battery includes techniques that assess auditory-motor organization, kinesthetic functions, higher visual functions, receptive and expressive language, reading and writing, arithmetic skill, memory, and intellectual processes. However, it is limited in the areas of attention and vigilance, visual memory, and nonverbal abstract reasoning. Its primary advantage is its ready adaptability to meet the needs of each individual case, but its lack of normative data restricts the valid interpretation of test results to very well-trained and highly experienced examiners. The use of Christensen's materials and especially Luria's approach and techniques cannot be considered a ready-to-use test battery in the sense of the usual psychometrically based approaches to assessment. Although very interesting and often useful in providing detailed information about an individual patient, any clinician interested in this approach must be thoroughly versed in Luria's philosophy, theories, and techniques, and must be prepared to design detailed single-subject experimental investigations for each patient.

Tests of General Cognitive Functioning

Wechsler Adult Intelligence Scale— Third Edition

The Wechsler Adult Intelligence Scale—Third Edition (WAIS-III)[47] is the current revision and restandardization of the familiar adult Wechsler intelligence scales. The test, which remains the standard for the clinical assessment of intelligence in patients between age 16 and age 89, provides data that quantify general intellectual functioning (Full-Scale IQ), verbal and nonverbal performance (Verbal and Performance Scale IQs), and specific performance in the areas of verbal-comprehension, perceptual-organization, working memory (attention), and processing speed. The Verbal Scale includes seven distinct subtests of verbally mediated cognitive functioning; the Performance Scale includes seven other subtests requiring visual-perceptual analysis, visual organization, comprehension, and psychomotor coordination. The summary IQ scores derived from the WAIS-III (and most other commonly used intelligence tests) have a normative mean of 100, with a standard deviation of 15.

Edith Kaplan introduced the WAIS-R as a Neuropsychological instrument,[22] which represents a synthesis of the process-oriented flexible assessment approach and a standard psychometric test of general cognitive functioning. After administration of the standard WAIS-R, this technique provides additional subtests, an alternate multiple-choice format for further assessment of the pattern and style of patients' functioning on a number of the subtests, a more comprehensive method of assessing specific deficits in arithmetic, and a new symbol copy task to better delineate the visuospatial processes involved in the standard Digit Symbol subtest. This allows a more comprehensive analysis of the nature of more specific cognitive processes underlying basic intelligence. The WAIS-RNI provides the means for a qualitative assessment of cognitive functioning in addition to the quantitative measure provided by the standard intelligence test.

Measures of Premorbid Intellectual Functioning

Interpretation of the clinical significance of neuropsychological findings for the individual patient depends in part on changes in functioning from premorbid levels. School records frequently contain the results of group tests of general ability (e.g., Otis-Lenon Test, Scholastic Aptitude Test, American College Test [ACT], and the like), which are useful for comparison purposes. Reports of school grades may also be used, although they tend to be less reliable. A number of techniques for estimating premorbid intellectual functioning from demographic information and test data gathered during the neuropsychological evaluation have been devised; including use of the Wechsler subtests of Vocabulary and Information, performance on tests of reading recognition (especially the National Adult Reading Test),[38] reliance on the patient's highest level of functioning on any test or set of tests, and the development of statistic regression equations based on demographic information. The use of demographic or psychometric variables to predict premorbid intelligence statistically has the advantages of using data readily generated during the neuropsychological evaluation, applying equally to virtually all patients, and not changing because of any clinical condition. Barona, Reynolds, and Chastain,[2] Krull et al.,[26] and others have developed and refined regression equations for predicting premorbid WAIS IQs at reasonably valid and reliable levels.

Tests of Attention and Vigilance
Digit Repetition

The number of digits repeated *forward* on the WAIS-III (or any other string of single-digit numbers) provides an easily administered objective measure of the patient's ability to maintain auditory attention for a brief period (approximately 10 to 15 seconds). The patient is verbally presented an increasing series of random digits at a rate of one digit per second (beginning with two digits and increasing until failure on two successive trials), and is requested to repeat the digit string exactly as heard.

Digits repeated *backward* requires very different mental processes, cognitively differing appreciably from digits repeated forward. Although attention is certainly *one* of the requirements of this task, it is far from the primary component of such performance; this task should therefore *not* be used to measure attention.

"A" Random Letter Test for Vigilance

This easily administered test of auditory attention is well described in Chapter 4.

Letter and Symbol Cancellation Tasks

Various visually presented letter, number, and symbol cancellation tasks can evaluate the patient's ability to maintain attention to visually presented stimuli for differing periods of time. These tasks typically include an array of randomly presented visual stimuli, with a given target item that must be noted and crossed out (e.g., letter, number, and symbol). The arrays presented by Mesulam[30] are particularly useful, as their format allows the examiner also to detect unilateral visual neglect and inattention.

Paced Auditory Serial Addition Test

The Paced Auditory Serial Addition Test (PASAT)[31] is a highly demanding and sensitive test of active sustained verbal attention, information processing, and basic ability to calculate. It consists of a taped series of randomized digit pairs that are presented at four different rates of speed, ranging from one digit every 1.2 seconds to one every 2.4 seconds. The patient is instructed to add each digit pair (e.g., "2–9 (11); 5–3 (8); 4–6 (10); 7–8 (15) . . ."). Derived scores include the percentage of correct responses at each rate, the total correct, and sometimes the mean time per correct response for each trial. New age-graded norms have been published recently, expanding the clinical usefulness of this test.[36]

Tests of Language Functioning

Peabody Picture Vocabulary Test—Third Edition

The Peabody Picture Vocabulary Test—Third Edition[9] is an easily administered test of single-word vocabulary comprehension. Norms are provided for age groups between $2\frac{1}{2}$ and 90 years. The test is composed of two equivalent 204-item word lists presented verbally in ascending order of difficulty. The patient responds by indicating which of four pictures best represents the word spoken by the examiner (e.g., "Where is 'incandescent'?"). The primary use of the Peabody test is as an objective test of spoken language at the single-word level, with an important secondary role of providing an early estimation of the patient's probable ability (or inability) to perform validly on both the language-mediated components of the neuropsychological evaluation and any other measure requiring language comprehension.

Token Test

The short version of the Token Test (see reference 44) is a well-structured, simply administered test of language comprehension that assesses the patient's ability to respond to various sentence types, semantic relations, and linguistic elements. The Token Test uses colored plastic tokens that are manipulated by the patient in response to a series of hierarchically ordered verbal commands (e.g., ranging from "Show me a circle" to "After touching the yellow square, pick up the blue triangle"). It is useful in the assessment of aphasic patients, as well as those with language comprehension deficits secondary to dementia, other neurologic conditions, or low levels of general intelligence.

Boston Naming Test

The Boston Naming Test (BNT)[23] is an objective measure of visual confrontation naming. It requires the patient to name a difficulty-graded series of pictured objects, ordered in increasing difficulty from "bed" to "abacus". When the patient is unable to spontaneously name an item, the examiner first provides a categorical cue (e.g., "It is something to eat" and then a phonemic cue (e.g., the beginning sound of the target word). Provisional norms are provided in the manual for children, normal adults, and aphasic adults;

additional norms derived from both normal and clinical samples are readily available.[43] Because of the frequent incidence of naming problems in various neurologic conditions, the BNT has deservedly become a very popular tool.

Verbal Fluency Tests

Several standardized tests of verbal fluency are currently available. The two that have proved most effective in our setting are the Controlled Oral Word-Association Test (FAS or CFL), adopted from the Multilingual Aphasia Examination—Third Edition (MAE—3),[4] and the Animal-Naming Test, adopted from the Boston Diagnostic Aphasia Examination (BDAE).[12] Both objectively measure the patient's ability spontaneously to produce single words under the restrictions of a limited category (e.g., "F") and time (60 seconds) (e.g., "Tell me all the words you can think of that begin with 'F' "). These tests are further discussed in Chapter 5. Updated norms for these procedures are available for a variety of age groups.[43]

Comprehensive Aphasia Batteries

When evaluating a patient with known aphasia or with a clinically apparent language obstacle to valid neuropsychological evaluation, a complete aphasia battery should be conducted. In some settings, this is the responsibility of the speech pathologist; in other instances, such batteries are administered by the neuropsychologist or behavioral neurologist. In either case, the clinician who deals with brain-damaged patients should be familiar with the contents, as well as the advantages and disadvantages, of the commonly used measures. The following is an alphabetic listing of the more popular batteries. Our preference is for the BDAE or the similar Western Aphasia Battery, although each of the listed tests has enjoyed considerable popularity.

- BDAE[12]
- Communication Abilities in Daily Living[19]
- MAE—3[4]
- Neurosensory Center Comprehensive Examination for Aphasia[43,44]
- Western Aphasia Battery[24]

See references 28 and 44 for reviews of the assessment process in aphasic patients and detailed descriptions of specific instruments.

Tests of Memory

Wechsler Memory Scale—Third Edition (WMS-III)

The publication of the Wechsler Memory Scale—Revised (WMS-R)[45] in 1987 and a subsequent reformulation and restandardization (WMS-III) in 1997[46] have provided neuropsychologists with a significant new omnibus measure of memory functioning. The WMS-R and -III are currently the most frequently used comprehensive measures of memory functioning in neuropsychological practice, although they have been criticized regarding their psychometric properties. The WMS-III includes a measure of general memory (actually composed of auditory and visual *delayed* recall), as well as indices of immediate memory (auditory and visual), working memory (auditory and visual), and auditory recognition (delayed). The WMS-R and -III are rather well standardized, with ample normative data provided in the test manuals and also available from numerous research studies for a wide range of age groups.

Memory Assessment Scales

The Memory Assessment Scales (MAS)[48] are a comprehensive battery for assessing memory functioning in adults. The MAS includes 12 subtests, based on seven learning and recall tasks, and provides summary scores for short-term memory (verbal span and visual span), verbal memory (word list recall and immediate recall of a logical paragraph), visual reproduction (15-second recall of visual designs and immediate visual recognition of visual designs), and global memory. The battery also includes methods to obtain verbal processing scores, measures of intrusion errors, and recognition memory. Although the MAS is psychometrically well designed and both clinically and theoretically interesting, clinical research data pertaining to this test are considerably more limited than for the more widely distributed WMS-R and -III.

Rey Auditory Verbal Learning Test; California Auditory Verbal Learning Test

The Rey Auditory Verbal Learning Test (RAVLT)[40] and the California Auditory Verbal Learning Test (CAVLT)[9] are easily administered tests of immediate verbal memory span, verbal learning, and immediate and delayed recall. In both tests word lists are verbally presented for five acquisition trials, requiring the patient to recall as many as possible of the verbally presented words after each trial. The tests provide a learning curve (presuming an increasing number of words recalled over successive trials) and document learning strategies (primacy or recency effects), retroactive and proactive interference, and intrusion errors, confusion, or confabulation tendencies. An interference trial followed by an immediate recall of the acquisition list and a short-term delayed recall provide retention scores. Recognition memory is assessed after the delayed recall trial. With additional delay trials (60 minutes, 24 hours, and so forth), the test can also measure verbal retention over more extended periods of time.

The CAVLT offers the advantage of using a word list that can be encoded by several different methods, allowing the examiner to further analyze learning and memory by measuring coding strategies, learning rates, other process data, and short- and long-term delay. Published norms and methods to statistically analyze the learning and recall processes are more sophisticated for the CAVLT than for the RAVLT. Neither test alone should be considered a sufficient test of all aspects of memory functioning, but both tests together are extremely useful for augmenting a more comprehensive memory assessment or for screening purposes.

Benton Visual Retention Test; Memory for Designs Test

The Benton Visual Retention Test (BVRT)[5,41] and the Memory for Designs (MFD) test[13] are measures designed to assess visual perception and analysis, short-term visual memory, and paper-and-pencil constructional ability. Each includes a series of graduated simple-to-complex line drawings that the patient must visually analyze and then copy. Both incorporate a memory component. The BVRT includes trials with variable periods of exposure of the stimuli as well as increasing periods of delay between exposure and reproduction, making it a more sensitive measure, albeit cognitively more complex. Both tests include explicit scoring instructions and adequate normative data. Because of its psychometric properties and its long history of research findings, most clinicians prefer the BVRT.

Tests of Abstraction and Higher Cognitive Function

Category Test

Among the tests of the Halstead-Reitan battery, many consider the Category Test[35] to be the most sensitive to the effects of brain dysfunction. The test consists of seven subtests of varying complexity, each with a different underlying principle (e.g., size, shape, color, and position). The patient is required to learn sorting behavior based on auditory or verbal reinforcement, and must also make conceptual shifts between categories upon reaching criteria for a given sorting strategy. Statistical studies suggest that the Category Test measures abstract reasoning and problem solving, conceptual set shifting, and the ability to learn from verbal reinforcement on tasks of moderate-level complexity. Category Test performance is related to age, education, and intelligence, at times resulting in interpretation problems when such variables are not taken into consideration. We have also noted problems caused by the effects of varying levels of attention and effort, as well as frustration and other emotional and behavioral factors. Newer, age-based norms[18] have proved helpful and should be used when this test is given. Short-form and paper-and-pencil versions of the test have been developed; we have found the Booklet Category Test,[7] which is more easily transported and administered in a hospital setting, to be a useful, valid, and reliable measure of higher-order conceptual functioning.

Wisconsin Card-Sorting Test

The Wisconsin Card-Sorting Test (WCST),[14] designed to assess abstract ability, conceptual set shifting, and "learning to learn," using tasks of medium-level complexity, was recently revised in terms of administration and scoring and has been subjected to a more refined standardization study.[18] The WCST requires the patient to sort a series of stimulus cards that vary in color, form, and number by matching to a sample array containing a red triangle, two green stars, three yellow crosses, and four blue circles. The examiner tells the patient whether his match is correct or incorrect after each trial. The designated "correct" matches are, in sequence: color—form—number—color—form—number. This test has received renewed clinical and research attention because (1) it provides an objective measure of abstraction and problem solving; (2) it is purported to be differentially sensitive to the effects of frontal lobe lesions (although this has certainly not been consistently found); and (3) it gives information on the particular reasons for difficulty on the test (e.g., impaired conceptualization, failure to sustain the correct set, perseveration, or deficits in learning across several trials). As with the Category Test, WCST results may be affected by the patient's general intelligence and academic background, as well as by emotional or behavioral factors; careful interpretation of results of each individual patient is therefore very important.

Raven's Progressive Matrices

Raven's Progressive Matrices[32–34] are a series of tests of visuospatial analysis, spatial conceptualization, and numeric reasoning. The test is available in three difficulty levels, ranging from the Coloured Matrices for children and impaired adults to the Advanced Matrices for well-functioning adults. Each of the test forms requires the patient to select, from a series of alternative possibilities, the pictured pattern or segment of a pattern that best matches or completes the stimulus figure. The matrices are useful for assessing visual pattern analysis, matching, nonverbal reasoning, unilateral neglect, and cognitive style. Additionally, the matrices can be used to differentiate between the visual analytic and the motor integration components in a patient who has documented "visual-perceptual deficits."

Tests of Sensory-Perceptual Functioning

Seashore Rhythm Test

This test of auditory perception and integration, an integral component of the Halstead-Reitan Battery and many of its derivatives, requires the patient to discriminate between pairs of recorded musical tones that are either identical ("same") or different. The Seashore Rhythm Test is primarily used within the Halstead-Reitan Battery to assess right temporal lobe functioning, although impaired performance may result also from more disparate or diffuse lesions. Varying attention levels, as well as basic difficulty in following directions, may adversely affect test performance, sometimes to the point of invalidating the results. Many neuropsychologists now consider the Seashore Rhythm Test to be a good test of auditory attention, notwithstanding its utility (or lack thereof) in localizing cerebral lesions.

Speech Sounds Perception Test

This subtest of the Halstead-Reitan Battery requires the patient to indicate on an answer sheet which one of four possible nonsense speech–like syllables he or she has heard via headphones (e.g., "heep ... **heet** ... wheep ... wheet"). The test includes 60 sets of syllables based on the vowel sound "ee," but beginning and ending with different consonants. Although it has been reported to be sensitive to the effects of brain damage, particularly left temporal lesions, considerable research suggests that it is primarily a measure of sustained attention. The examiner who wishes to use the test for its original purpose must ensure that sufficient basic attention was maintained over the course of the administration to allow valid interpretation of the higher-level component of the test. Once again, behavioral and emotional problems can have an adverse effect on test performance, causing invalid results.

Tests of Tactile Perception

A variety of objective tests of tactile suppression, tactile recognition (stereognosis), and graphesthesia (e.g., fingertip writing recognition, palm writing) have been developed to assess unilateral parietal lobe functioning. With the exception of normative data for objective comparison, the measures are very similar to clinical tests conducted during the standard neurologic and extended mental status examination.

Tests of Visual Perception

It is crucial to establish the adequacy of the patient's visual acuity and visual perception and to rule out the possibility of unilateral neglect or inattention. Much of this is accomplished using clinical methods identical to those used in the standard neurologic examination. Tests of neglect, color vision, visual recognition, facial recognition, fragmented visual stimuli,[20] and figure-ground discrimination are merely examples of the many standardized tests and procedures that can be used to assess these functions. See references 28 and 44 for reviews of available measures.

Tests of Constructional Ability
Bender Gestalt Test

The Bender Gestalt Test (originally the Bender Visual Motor Gestalt[3]) is a venerable, rapidly administered screening test of paper-and-pencil constructional ability. The patient is presented with a series of simple and more difficult geometric line drawings, which are copied. The patient's design reproductions can be objectively scored for the errors of integration, distortion, perseveration, and rotation.[25] Unfortunately, this test is still used fairly commonly as a screening measure for "organicity." This use is unwarranted given the current state of knowledge regarding brain-behavior relationships. It is quite appropriate to include it as a test of one type of constructional ability within the context of a more comprehensive battery, however.

Raven's Progressive Matrices

These tests are useful in assessing the visuospatial analytic component of the constructional process.

Benton Visual Retention Test

This well-standardized test can also be used to evaluate both reproduction constructional ability (design copying) and short-term recall reproduction (constructions from memory). The major advantages of this test are standard administration and scoring criteria, good normative and research data, and the availability of alternate, equivalent test forms.

Hooper Visual Organization Test

The Hooper Visual Organization Test (HVOT)[20] has recently gained renewed favor in neuropsychology as a measure of visual analysis and organization and of the ability to synthesize disparate arts into a meaningful gestalt without a motor component. The test includes a series of line drawings of increasing complexity that have been cut into a variety of separate parts. The patient must identify the pictured object by mentally organizing the various parts. The HVOT is essentially a "constructional" test without a motor-output component. In addition to the patient's absolute level of performance, the HVOT is useful in demonstrating the more specific underlying nature of a patient's perceptual motor dysfunction.

Tests of Visual Motor Sequencing
Trail-Making Test

This test, which is included in the Halstead-Reitan Battery, is a popular measure of visual searching, visual sequencing, perceptuomotor speed, the ability to make alternating conceptual shifts efficiently, and attention. Part A of the test merely requires the patient to draw a line sequencing the numbers 1 through 25. Part B includes an element of conceptual shifting, requiring the sequencing of numbers and letters in alternating fashion (e.g., 1–A–2–B–3–C–4 . . .). Both speed and accuracy are considered in the interpretation of this test. Currently available research shows that this test (particularly Part B) is sensitive to the effects of brain dysfunction of any type and also provides some equivocal indication that patients with frontal lobe lesions perform relatively more poorly than those with lesions in other loci.

Digit Symbol Modalities

The Digit Symbol Modalities (DSM) test,[42] essentially a symbol coding task under timed conditions, assesses visual scanning, visual tracking (attention), and psychomotor speed. The patient is presented with a printed key associating the numbers 1 through 9 with a different symbol, and a test form containing an array of 110 blank squares, each paired with a random symbol. The patient then writes as many numbers under the correct symbol as possible within a 90-second time span. The DSM test also includes a verbally presented component, which allows a comparison between the accuracy and speed of written and oral responses. The test requires sustained attention, visual search, visual sequencing, and learning ability. DSM test performance is sensitive to the effects of central nervous system dysfunction and appears to be related to real-world functioning.[44]

Tests of Motor Coordination and Strength

Finger-Tapping Test

The Finger-Tapping Test, also known as the Finger Oscillation Test, is a frequently used measure of upper extremity motor speed. The test includes a number of tapping trials by the index finger of each hand using a mechanical or electrical recording tapping device. A number of reports suggest an average for normal subjects of approximately 55 taps with the dominant hand during a 10-second trial and approximately 10% fewer with the nondominant hand. The test is somewhat sensitive to anterior brain dysfunction in general and, more specifically, to lesions in the area of the contralateral motor strip.

Grooved Pegboard

The Grooved Pegboard[29] is a very useful measure of upper extremity speed, combined with manipulatory dexterity. Patients must rapidly place ridged pegs in a board containing a series of randomly grooved holes, using first the dominant hand alone and then the nondominant hand alone. Because of the presence of randomly positioned slots, the test is more complex and accordingly more sensitive than most pegboards. It is a good tool to objectify more subtle motor deficits and to assess improvements in hand coordination following stroke or trauma. A wide range of standardized norms, as well as mean scores from various clinical samples, are available to aid in the interpretation of the test results.

Hand Dynamometer (Grip Strength)

The use of a mechanical hand dynamometer to assess grip strength over several (usually five) trials with the right and left hands allows the accurate quantification of a common motor component of the standard neurologic examination. Reductions in strength bilaterally when compared with the expected levels for age and sex, as well as disproportionate discrepancies between hands, may indicate brain dysfunction, particularly when peripheral factors are ruled out.

Tests of Academic Achievement

Wide-Range Achievement Test— Third Edition

The Wide-Range Achievement Test—Third Edition (WRAT-III)[49] is probably the most frequently used objective screening test of achievement, owing partly to its brevity. It assesses performance in reading recognition (reading isolated words graduated in difficulty), spelling to dictation (using words ranging from kindergarten to high-school level), and computational arithmetic (ranging from simple counting to addition, subtraction, division, multiplication, and algebraic formulas). Norms allow comparison of the individual patient's performance with normal samples ranging from 5 to 75 years of age and educational levels from preschool to grade 12.[8]

Woodcock-Johnson Psychoeducational Battery—Revised: Tests of Achievement

The Woodcock-Johnson Psychoeducational Battery—Revised: Tests of Achievement (WJ-R-Ach)[50] represents a wide–age-range measure of academic achievement in the basic areas of reading, mathematics, and written language, as well as in elementary science, social studies, and humanities. Neuropsychological studies usually focus on the three basic areas. A major advantage of this battery is the incorporation of supplemental subtests that allow the evaluation of specific deficits within the basic areas. The WJ-R-Ach is well developed psychometrically and is also well standardized; it offers a more comprehensive measure of academic functioning than most of the commonly used screening tests and is useful when evaluating patients with primary learning disorders or acquired academic deficits.

Personality Tests

Minnesota Multiphasic Personality Inventory–2

The recently revised Minnesota Multiphasic Personality Inventory–2 (MMPI-2)[16] continues to be the most commonly used standardized test of emotional status in both psychiatric and neurologic patients. By comparing each patient's performance with those of normal individuals, the MMPI-2 measures emotional status in the areas of hypochondriasis (physical concern), depression, hysteria (reduced ability to cope and tendency to channel emotional stress into somatic outlets), personality disorder (or chronicity), masculinity-femininity of interests, paranoia, psychasthenia (anxiety and obsessive-compulsive traits), schizophrenia (or cognitive confusion), hypomania (agitation), and social introversion. In addition to the 10 basic clinical scales, the MMPI-2 provides 15 new content scales, offering a much more comprehensive description of the patient's emotional functioning.

At our current state of knowledge and experience with this technique, the MMPI-2 is considered more appropriate for assessing normal individuals and psychiatric patients than for brain-damaged patients. However, the literature pertaining to the use of the MMPI with brain-damaged patients is expanding; the reviews by Lezak[28] and Spreen and Strauss[44] are good introductions. See also Algano and colleagues[1] for a recent study of MMPI use in investigating the emotional changes that occur after closed-head injury. Despite some contention regarding the nature of interpretations of MMPI abnormalities within the context of neurologic disease, it continues to be most useful in *describing* emotional functioning in neurologic patients, rather than in establishing a psychiatric diagnosis in accordance with the *Diagnostic and Statistical Manual of Mental Disorders—Fourth Edition (DSM-IV)*.

Other Personality Instruments

A variety of self-reporting scales of anxiety, depression, physical symptoms, more specific neurobehavioral symptoms, pain and its social ramifications, and social adjustment are available for use with patients who are capable of responding validly either in written form or during an interview. Such tests can be useful for assessing the patient's subjective perception of emotional and social well-being, as well as for research purposes. See Lezak[28] and Spreen and Strauss[44] for more information regarding these instruments.

REFERENCES

1. Algano, DP, et al: The MMPI and closed-head injury. Clin Neuropsychol. 6:134, 1992.
2. Barona, A, Reynolds, CR, and Chastain, R: A demographically based index of pre-morbid intelligence of the WAIS-R. J Consult Clin Psychol 52:885, 1984.
3. Bender, L: Bender Motor Gestalt Test. American Orthopsychiatric Association, New York, 1946.
4. Benton, AL, deS Hamsher, K, and Silven, AB: Multilingual Aphasia Examination, ed 3. AJA Associates, Iowa City, 1983.
5. Benton, AL, et al: Contributions to Neuropsychological Assessment: A Clinical Manual. Oxford University Press, New York, 1994.
6. Christensen, AL: Luria's Neuropsychological Investigation, ed 2. Western Psychological Services, Los Angeles, 1979.
7. DeFilippis, NA and McCampbell, MS: The Booklet Category Test. Psychological Assessment Resources, Odessa, FL, 1987.
8. Delise, DC, et al: California Verbal Learning Test. Psychological Corporation, San Antonio, 1987.
9. Dunn, LM and Dunn, LM: Peabody Picture Vocabulary Test, ed 3. American Guidance Service, Circle Pines, MN, 1997.
10. Golden, CJ, Purisch, AD, and Hammeke, TA: Luria Nebraska Neuropsychological Battery: Forms I and II. Western Psychological Services, Los Angeles, 1986.
11. Goldstein, G and Incagnoli, TM: Contemporary Approaches to Neuropsychological Assessment. Plenum Press, New York, 1998.
12. Goodglass, H and Kaplan, E: The Assessment of Aphasia and Related Disorders. Lea & Febiger, Philadelphia, 1983.
13. Graham, FK and Kendall, BS: Memory-for-Designs Test: Revised General Manual. Percept Mot Skills (Suppl 2-VIII)11:147, 1960.
14. Grant, DA and Berg, EA: Wisconsin Card Sorting Test. Psychologic Corporation, San Antonio, 1993.
15. Halstead, W: Brain and Intelligence: A Qualitative Study of the Frontal Lobes. University of Chicago Press, Chicago, 1947.
16. Hathaway, SR, et al: Minnesota Multiphasic Personality Inventory–2: Manual for Administration and Scoring. University of Minnesota Press, Minneapolis, 1989.
17. Heaton, RK: Wisconsin Card Sorting Test Manual. Psychological Assessment Resources, Odessa, FL, 1981.
18. Heaton, RK, Grant, I, and Matthews, CG: Comprehensive Norms for an Expanded Halstead-Reitan Battery. Psychological Assessment Resources, Odessa, FL, 1991.
19. Holland, AL: Communicative Abilities in Daily Living. University Park Press, Baltimore, 1980.
20. Hooper, HE: The Hooper Visual Organization Test. Western Psychological Services, Los Angeles, 1958.
21. Jarvis, PE and Barth, JT: The Halstead-Reitan Neuropsychological Battery: A Guide to Interpretation and Clinical Applications. Psychological Assessment Resources, Odessa, FL, 1994.
22. Kaplan, E: WAIS-R as a Neuropsychological Instrument. Psychological Corporation, San Antonio, 1991.
23. Kaplan, E, Goodglass, H, and Weintraub, S: Boston Naming Test. Lea & Febiger, Philadelphia, 1983.
24. Kertesz, A: Aphasia and Related Disorders: Taxonomy, Localization, and Recovery. Grune & Stratton, New York, 1982.
25. Koppitz, EM: The Bender Gestalt Test for Young Children. Grune & Stratton, New York, 1963.
26. Krull, KR, Scott, JG, and Sherer, M: Estimation of premorbid intelligence from combined performance and demographic variables. The Clinical Neuropsychologist 9:83, 1995.
27. Lees-Hailey, PR, et al: Forensic neuropsychological test usage: An empirical survey. Archives of Clinical Neuropsychology 11:45, 1995.
28. Lezak, MD: Neuropsychologic Assessment, ed 3. Oxford University Press, New York, 1995.
29. Matthews, CG and Klove, H: Instruction Manual for the Adult Neuropsychology Test Battery. University of Wisconsin Medical School, Madison, WI, 1964.
30. Mesulam, M-M: Principles of Behavioral Neurology: Tests of Directed Attention and Memory. FA Davis, Philadelphia, 1985.

31. Psychological Corporation: Paced Auditory Serial Addition Test. Psychological Corporation, San Antonio, 1994.
32. Raven, JC: Guide to the Standard Progressive Matrices. Psychological Corporation, San Antonio, 1977.
33. Raven, JC: Guide to Using the Coloured Progressive Matrices. Psychological Corporation, San Antonio, 1977.
34. Raven, JC: The Advanced Progressive Matrices. Psychological Corporation, San Antonio, 1977.
35. Reitan, RM and Wolfson, D: The Halstead-Reitan Neuropsychological Test Battery: Theory and Clinical Interpretation, ed 2. Neuropsychology Press, Tucson, AZ, 1993.
36. Roman, DD, et al: Extended norms for the Paced Serial Addition Test. The Clinical Neuropsychologist 5:33, 1991.
37. Russell, EW, Neuringer, C, and Goldstein, G: Assessment of Brain Damage: A Neuropsychological Key Approach. Wiley-Interscience, New York, 1970.
38. Ryan, JJ and Paolo, AM: A screening procedure for estimating premorbid intelligence in the elderly. Clin Neuropsychol 6:53, 1992.
39. Sbordone, RJ and Long, CJ (Eds): Ecological Validity of Neuropsychological Testing. GR Press/St Lucie Press, Delray Beach, FL, 1996.
40. Schmidt, M: Manual for the Rey Auditory Verbal Learning Test. Western Psychological Services, Los Angeles, 1997.
41. Sivan, AB: Benton Visual Retention Test, ed 5. Psychological Corporation, San Antonio, 1992.
42. Smith, A: Symbol Digit Modalities Test. Western Psychological Services, Los Angeles, 1991.
43. Spreen, O and Benton, AL: Neurosensory Center Comprehensive Examination for Aphasia. University of Victoria Neuropsychology Laboratory, Victoria, BC, 1977.
44. Spreen, O and Strauss, E: A Compendium of Neuropsychological Tests, ed 2. Oxford University Press, New York, 1998.
45. Wechsler, D: Wechsler Memory Scale—Revised (WMS-R). Psychological Corporation, San Antonio, 1987.
46. Wechsler, D: Wechsler Memory Scale—Third Edition (WMS-III). Psychological Corporation, San Antonio, 1997.
47. Wechsler, D: Wechsler Adult Intelligence Scale—Third Edition (WAIS-III). Psychological Corporation, San Antonio, 1997.
48. Williams, MJ: Memory Assessment Scales (MAS). Psychological Assessment Resources. Odessa, FL, 1991.
49. Wilkinson, GS: The Wide Range Achievement Test—Third Edition. Jastak Associates, Wilmington, DE, 1993.
50. Woodcock, RW and Mather, N: Woodcock-Johnson Tests of Achievement. DLM Teaching Resources, Allen, TX, 1989.

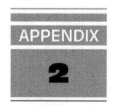

MENTAL STATUS EXAMINATION RECORDING FORM

PATIENT INFORMATION

Patient name: Date:
Address: Case #:

Phone: Hospital #:
Date of birth: Place of birth:
Age: Sex:
Education:
   Highest level: Age at completion:
   Failures or honors:
Handedness:
   Patient: Family:
Occupation:
Medical diagnosis:
   Onset and nature:

Hemiplegia:
   (Circle)   None   Recovered   Right   Left

Hemianopia:
   (Circle)   None   Recovered   Right   Left

Neurosurgical information:

Electroencephalograph (EEG) focus:

MRI, CT scan, brain scan, angiogram, and so forth:

(Starred items should be used with all patients.)

*I. Behavioral Observations

*A. History of behavior change, memory difficulties, bizarre behavior, change in work habits, and the like:

*B. Physical Appearance:

*C. Emotional Status (e.g., confusion, depression, anxiety, lability):

 D. Frontal Lobe Test Results (see related cortical functions):

*E. Denial or Neglect:

*II. Level of Consciousness

*A. Rate: Alert_____ Lethargic_____ Stupor_____ Coma_____

*B. Describe stimulus necessary to arouse patient, and record patient's response:

*III. Attention

*A. Observation of patient during examination:

*B. Digit repetition: Repeat digits at a rate of one per second.

Item	Check If Correct
3–7	_____
2–4–9	_____
8–5–2–7	_____
2–9–6–8–3	_____
5–7–1–9–4–6	_____
8–1–5–9–3–6–2	_____
3–9–8–2–5–1–4–7	_____
7–2–8–5–4–6–7–3–9	_____

C. Vigilance: Repeat letters at a rate of one per second. Tell patient to indicate by tapping the table whenever he or she hears the letter "A."

```
L T P E  A O A I  C T  D A L  A A
A N I  A B F  S A M R  Z E O A D
P A K L  A U C J  T  O E  A B  A A
Z Y K M U S  A H E  V  A A R  A T
```

1. Errors of omission: _____
2. Errors of commission: _____

D. Unilateral inattention:

*IV. Language

*A. Spontaneous speech:

  *1. Describe, including fluency, articulation, and presence of paraphasias:
  2. Verbal fluency: Total animals: _____
  Total words: _____

*B. Comprehension:

  *1. Patient's response to pointing commands:
  Ask patient to point to one, two, three, then four room objects or body parts in sequence. Record adequacy of performance.

  *2. Patient's response to yes-no questions:
  (e.g., "Is it raining today?" or "Is Grant still president?")

*C. Repetition:

  Tell the patient to repeat each of the following:

Item	Check If Correct
1. Ball	_____
2. Help	_____
3. Airplane	_____
4. Hospital	_____
5. Mississippi River	_____
6. The little boy went home.	_____
7. We all went over there together.	_____

Item	Check If Correct
8. The old car wouldn't start on Tuesday morning.	_____
9. The short fat boy dropped the china vase.	_____
10. Each fight readied the boxer for the championship bout.	_____

*D. Naming and Word Finding:

Tell the patient to name the following simple colors and objects:

Item	Check If Correct
1. Colors	
a. Red	_____
b. Blue	_____
c. Yellow	_____
d. Pink	_____
e. Purple	_____
2. Body parts	
a. Eye	_____
b. Leg	_____
c. Teeth	_____
d. Thumb	_____
e. Knuckles	_____
3. Clothing and room objects	
a. Door	_____
b. Watch	_____
c. Shoe	_____
d. Shirt	_____
e. Ceiling	_____
4. Parts of objects	
a. Watch stem (winder)	_____
b. Coat lapel	_____
c. Watch crystal	_____
d. Sole of shoe	_____
e. Buckle of belt	_____

E. Reading:

Describe level of adequacy (words, sentences, paragraphs) and note types of errors:

F. Writing:

Describe level of adequacy and note types of errors:

G. Spelling:

Describe performance to dictation and note errors:

*V. Memory

Most of the following memory tasks evaluate verbal memory. In patients with language disturbance (aphasia), the visual memory tests must be used.

*A. Immediate Recall (short-term memory):
Refer to Digit Repetition in Section III.

*B. Orientation:

	Check If Correct
*1. Person	
a. Name	_____
b. Age	_____
c. Birth date	_____
*2. Place	
a. Location (at present)	_____
b. City location	_____
c. Home address	_____
*3. Time	
a. Date	_____
b. Day of the week	_____
c. Time of day	_____
d. Season of the year	_____
e. Duration of time with examiner	_____

C. Remote Memory:

	Check If Correct or Adequate
*1. Personal Information	
a. Where were you born?	_____
b. School information	_____
c. Vocational history	_____
d. Family information	_____

**Check If Correct
or Adequate**

*2. Historic Facts
   a. Four US presidents during   _____
      your lifetime
   b. Last war   _____

*D. New-Learning Ability:

   1. Four Unrelated Words: Tell the patient, "I am going to tell you
      four words, which I want you to remember." Have the patient
      repeat the four words after they are initially presented and
      then say that you will ask him or her to remember the words
      later. Continue with the examination, and at intervals of 5,
      10, and 30 minutes, ask the patient to recall the words. Use
      categoric ("one word is a color") or phonemic ("one word
      begins with B") cues if he or she is unable to recall the word
      spontaneously on any trial. Record the type and amount of
      cuing necessary. Three alternate sets of words are provided.

	5 min	10 min	30 min
a. Brown (Fun) (Grape)	____	____	____
b. Honesty (Loyalty) (Happiness)	____	____	____
c. Tulip (Carrot) (Stocking)	____	____	____
d. Eyedropper (Ankle) (Toothbrush)	____	____	____

Describe type of cues used if necessary:

   2. Verbal Story for Immediate Recall:
      Tell the patient, "I am going to read you a short story, which
      I want you to remember. Listen closely to what I read be-
      cause I will ask you to tell me the story when I finish." Read
      the story slowly and carefully, but without pausing at the
      slash marks. After completing the paragraph, tell the patient
      to retell the story as accurately as possible. Record the num-
      ber of correct memories (information within the slashes)
      and describe confabulation if it is present.

It was July / and the Rogers / had packed up / their four children
/ in the station wagon / and were off / on vacation.

They were taking / their yearly trip / to the beach / at Gulf Shores.

This year / they were making / a special / one-day stop / at the
Aquarium / in New Orleans.

After a long day's drive / they arrived / at the motel / only to
discover / that in their excitement / they had left / the twins /
and their suitcases / in the front yard.

a. Number of correct memories: _____

b. Describe confabulation if present:

3. Visual Memory (hidden objects):

Tell the patient that you are going to hide some objects around the office, desk, or bed and that you want him or her to remember where they are. Hide four or five common objects (e.g., keys, pen, reflex hammer) in various areas in the patient's sight. After a delay of several minutes, ask the patient to find the objects. Ask patient to name those items he or she is unable to find.

a. Number of hidden objects found: _____

b. Number of hidden objects named but not found: _____

c. Number of locations indicated but objects not named: _____

4. Paired Associated Learning:

Tell the patient that you are going to read a list of words two at a time. The patient will be expected to remember the words that go together (e.g., big—little). When he or she is clear as to the directions, read the first list of words at the rate of one pair per second. After reading the first list, test for recall by presenting the first recall list. Give the first word of a pair and ask for the word that went with it. Correct incorrect responses and proceed to the next pair. After the first recall has been completed, allow a 10-second delay and continue with the second presentation and recall lists.

PRESENTATION LISTS	
1	**2**
a. Weather—Box	a. House—Income
b. High—Low	b. Weather—Box
c. House—Income	c. Book—Page
d. Book—Page	d. High—Low

RECALL LISTS	
1	**2**
a. House _____	a. High _____
b. High _____	b. House _____
c. Weather _____	c. Book _____
d. Book _____	d. Weather _____

1. Number of easy paired associates recalled: _____

2. Number of difficult paired associates recalled: _____

*VI. Constructional Ability

*A. Reproduction drawings:
Ask the patient to copy the following drawings in the space provided.

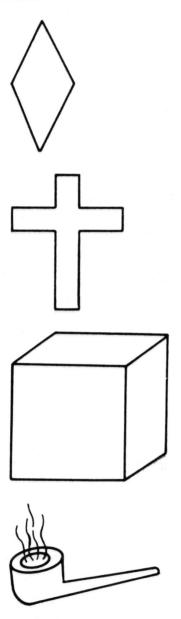

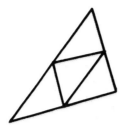

Item	Score
1. Vertical diamond	_____
2. Two-dimensional cross	_____
3. Three-dimensional cube	_____
4. Three-dimensional pipe	_____
5. Triangle within a triangle	_____

Total score: _____

*B. Drawings to Command:
Tell the patient to draw the following pictures in the space provided.

Clock with all numbers
Set clock for 2:30 or 5 to 3.

Daisy in flowerpot

House in perspective

Item	Score
1. Clock	_____
2. Daisy in flowerpot	_____
3. House in perspective	_____

Total score: _____

C. Block Designs:

(See stimulus cards)

Item	Score
1. Design 1	_____
2. Design 2	_____
3. Design 3	_____
4. Design 4	_____

Total score: _____

Describe types of errors:

*VII. Higher Cognitive Functions

A. Fund of Information:

Item	Check If Correct
1. How many weeks are in a year?	_____
2. Why do people have lungs?	_____
3. Name four US Presidents since 1940.	_____
4. Where is Denmark?	_____
5. How far is it from New York to Los Angeles?	_____
6. Why are light colored clothes cooler in the summer than dark colored clothes?	_____
7. What is the capital of Spain?	_____
8. What causes rust?	_____
9. Who wrote the Odyssey?	_____
10. What is the Acropolis?	_____

Total score: _____

*B. Calculations:
Describe the patient's adequacy in performance and types of errors made on the following types of calculations:

1. Verbal rote examples:

a. Addition	$(4 + 6)$
b. Subtraction	$(8 - 5)$
c. Multiplication	(2×8)
d. Division	$(56 \div 8)$

2. Verbal complex examples:

a. Addition   (14 + 17)
b. Subtraction   (43 − 38)
c. Multiplication   (21 × 5)
d. Division   (128 ÷ 8)

*3. Written complex examples:

a. Addition
$$\begin{array}{r} 108 \\ +\ 79 \\ \hline \end{array}$$

b. Subtraction
$$\begin{array}{r} 605 \\ -\ 86 \\ \hline \end{array}$$

c. Multiplication
$$\begin{array}{r} 108 \\ \times\ 36 \\ \hline \end{array}$$

d. Division $43\overline{)559}$

*C. Proverb Interpretation:
Tell the patient to explain the following sayings. Record the answers.

Item	Score
1. Don't cry over spilled milk.	_____
2. Rome wasn't built in a day.	_____
3. A drowning man will clutch at a straw.	_____

4. A golden hammer can break down an
   iron door.   _____

5. The hot coal burns; the cold one
   blackens.   _____

   Total score: _____
   Total concrete responses: _____

*D. Similarities

Item	Score
1. Turnip .... Cauliflower	_____
2. Car .... Airplane	_____
3. Desk .... Bookcase	_____
4. Poem .... Novel	_____
5. Horse .... Apple	_____

   Total score: _____
   Total concrete responses: _____

VIII. Related Cortical Functions

A. Ideomotor Apraxia:
   Describe the adequacy of the patient's performance in carrying out
   motor acts to command using buccofacial, limb, and whole body
   commands. Indicate if imitation or use of the real object was necessary to facilitate performance.

Item	Score
1. Blow out a match.	_____
2. Drink through a straw.	_____
3. Lick crumbs off your lips.	_____
4. Comb your hair.	_____
5. Flip a coin.	_____

B. Ideational Apraxia:
   Describe the adequacy of the patient's performance on the following complex motor tasks:

   1. Letter-envelope-stamp
   2. Candle-holder-match
   3. Toothpaste-toothbrush

C. Psychomotor speed (if indicated):

Ask patient to write the letters of the alphabet in
capitals.   **Time in**
                                                         Seconds

                                                         _____

D. Right-Left Disorientation:

Item	**Check If Correct**
1. Identification on self	_____
a. Show me your right foot	_____
b. Show me your left hand	_____
2. Crossed commands on self	_____
a. With your right hand touch your left shoulder.	_____
b. With your left hand touch your right ear.	_____
3. Identification on examiner	_____
a. Point to my left knee.	_____
b. Point to my right elbow.	_____
4. Crossed commands on examiner	_____
a. With your right hand point to my left eye.	_____
b. With your left hand point to my left foot.	_____

Describe nature and degree of errors made:

E. Finger Agnosia:
Describe the adequacy of the patient's nonverbal and verbal
performance.

F. Gerstmann's Syndrome:
Describe the nature and degree of impairment in the following
areas if present in the patient:

1. Finger agnosia: _____
2. Right-left disorientation: _____
3. Dysgraphia: _____
4. Dyscalculia: _____

G. Visual Agnosia:
Describe any deficits in visual identification of objects, naming of objects whose use can be demonstrated, color naming, and facial recognition:

H. Astereognosis:
Describe deficits:

Left hand _____
Right hand _____

I. Geographic Disorientation:

1. Describe evidence of disorientation obtained from history:

2. Map localization:
Describe patient's ability to localize well-known cities on a map:

3. Orientation of self in hospital:
Describe patient's ability to orient self within the hospital environment:

*J. Denial and Neglect:

	Yes	No
If present, describe patient's response.		
1. Does patient frankly deny his illness?	_____	_____
2. Is there evidence of unilateral neglect? (e.g., shaving one side of face, dressing one arm, and so on)	_____	_____
3. Is there evidence of unilateral neglect on drawings? (e.g., absence of numbers on one side of clock or absence of one side of picture)	_____	_____

K. Frontal Lobe Tests:

1. Drawings:
   Tell the patient to copy and continue the following sequence. Record evidence of perservation or loss of sequence.

   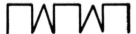

2. Alternating hand sequences:
   This is a motor alternation task that uses both hands. Initially, the patient places both hands on the desk, one in a fist and one with the fingers extended palm down. Tell the patient to alternate the position of the two hands rapidly (simultaneously extending the fingers of one hand while making a fist with the other). Record if the patient is unable to maintain the alternating sequence.

SUMMARY OF FINDINGS

1. Describe major areas of impairment:

2. Tentative neurobehavioral diagnosis:

3. Tentative localization:

4. Tentative clinical diagnosis:

5. Proposed management plans:

INDEX

Page numbers followed by *f* indicate figures; those followed by *t* indicate tables.